FEATURES

WINTER 2023 • NUMBER 34

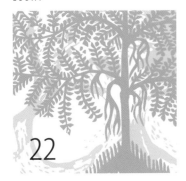
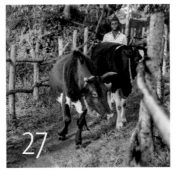
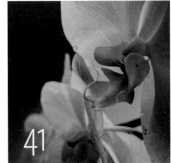
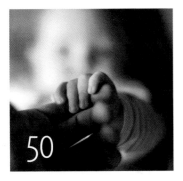
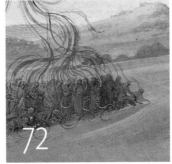
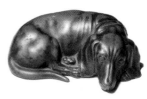

Plough

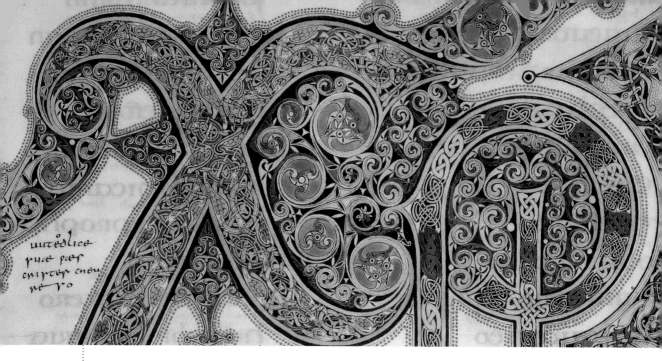

uuредісса
руає раоу
спірує споu
nt̃ vo

DEPARTMENTS

WEB EXCLUSIVES

Read these articles at *plough.com/web34*.

Plough

ANOTHER LIFE IS POSSIBLE

EDITOR: Peter Mommsen
SENIOR EDITORS: Maureen Swinger, Sam Hine, Susannah Black Roberts
EDITOR-AT-LARGE: Caitrin Keiper
MANAGING EDITOR: Maria Hine
BOOKS AND CULTURE EDITOR: Joy Marie Clarkson
POETRY EDITOR: A. M. Juster
DESIGNERS: Rosalind Stevenson, Miriam Burleson
CREATIVE DIRECTOR: Clare Stober
COPY EDITORS: Wilma Mommsen, Priscilla Jensen
FACT CHECKER: Suzanne Quinta
MARKETING DIRECTOR: Trevor Wiser
UK EDITION: Ian Barth
CONTRIBUTING EDITORS: Leah Libresco Sargeant, Brandon McGinley, Jake Meador
FOUNDING EDITOR: Eberhard Arnold (1883–1935)

Plough Quarterly No. 34: Generations
Published by Plough Publishing House, ISBN 978-1-63608-074-1
Copyright © 2023 by Plough Publishing House. All rights reserved.

EDITORIAL OFFICE
151 Bowne Drive
Walden, NY 12586
T: 845.572.3455
info@plough.com

SUBSCRIBER SERVICES
PO Box 8542
Big Sandy, TX 75755
T: 800.521.8011
subscriptions@plough.com

United Kingdom
Brightling Road
Robertsbridge
TN32 5DR
T: +44(0)1580.883.344

Australia
4188 Gwydir Highway
Elsmore, NSW
2360 Australia
T: +61(0)2.6723.2213

Plough Quarterly (ISSN 2372-2584) is published quarterly by
Plough Publishing House, PO Box 398, Walden, NY 12586.

Individual subscription $36 / £24 / €28 per year.
Subscribers outside of the United States and Canada pay in British pounds or euros.

Periodicals postage paid at Walden, NY 12586 and at additional mailing offices.

POSTMASTER: Send address changes to
Plough Quarterly, PO Box 8542, Big Sandy, TX 75755.

Front cover: Hung Liu, *Tobacco Sharecroppers*, archival pigment print with hand work and gold leafing, 2017. Courtesy of Hung Liu Studios and Gail Severn Gallery.

Back cover: Shonto Begay, *Tree of Seven Hearts*, acrylic on canvas, 2014. Used by permission from the artist and Tom Alexander Photography.

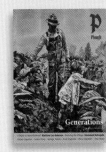

ABOUT THE COVER

A father passes his knowledge of plants and farming down to his young daughter. This image gives artistic voice to the skills and wisdom we can learn from older generations and in turn pass down to the next. Artwork by Chinese-American artist Hung Liu (1948–2021).

LETTERS

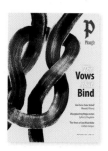

Readers respond to *Plough*'s Autumn 2022 issue, "The Vows that Bind." Send letters to *letters@plough.com.*

LASTING RELATIONSHIPS

On Peter Mommsen's "Word Is Bond": A timely article that we all should mull over. We live in a world of instant gratification without thought of the dangerous consequences that follow. In our modern world, anything goes – there's a passion for more and more excitement. How on earth can one expect to have peace within oneself or spread that much-needed peace in the world if the foundations for a lasting relationship are not properly laid in the first place? Today, one can divorce on the flimsiest of excuses. The divorce rates, even in countries where once there was a strong Christian faith, are on the increase. Cohabiting is considered the new "marriage" even though separations in such unions continue to rise. The simple answer to this chaos is genuine repentance and a return to God.

Mervyn Maciel, Sutton, Surrey, England

TRUE FREEDOM

On Wendell Berry's "Can Love Take Sides?": Berry's insights about what happens when those who aim to take "the side of love" start hating the haters strike a strong chord with me. In a way, it's a good telling of the alternative to Martin Luther King's "double victory" of wearing down hate with love: the alternative is being overcome by hate (and thus becoming *what* we hate).

One closing point I take some issue with, following a thread woven through much of Berry's writing, is the dichotomy of settlers and exploiters, set up as opposites. It's clear that by "settlers" he means people who love and care for a particular place, but it bears reminding that pioneers and colonists have also been settlers in a more malevolent sense – seeking new lands, yes, but then settling in places in order to exploit them. And many hunter-gatherer and pastoral societies have lived nomadically in much less exploitative ways. So have some who have followed calls to service in places where they might live more simply than they could perhaps have chosen, swimming against the current of a dehumanizing economy.

This is not to take an exact opposite position to Berry's that settlers are bad and nomads are good, but rather that no such neat parallel exists: exploitative behaviors can be found among both sedentaries and nomads, as can caring behaviors. I may have to give more thought to what the opposite of "exploiter" might be, but "settler" is not it. Carer, maybe?

Julia Smucker, Biddeford, Maine

Berry is always a champion for the oppressed and needy. I'd like to see *Plough* broaden its understanding of those who are oppressed and enslaved to include those trapped with addictions, including to social media – there is so much science showing social media is a trap of enslavement and addiction. Dr. Leonard Sax is one voice of many highlighting the brain damage associated with overuse of social media and porn. Perhaps *Plough* can do a deep dive on this evil trap, how it enslaves and how people can become free and return to their right minds.

Steve Knudtsen, Broomfield, Colorado

WHEN WE ARE SENT

On Norann Voll's "The Adventure of Obedience": Beautifully written devotional article. Deeply moving and convicting. When I joined my church twenty-six years ago, it also required vows. At first, I hesitated, but God showed me that as a single woman I needed to experience and understand what faithfulness looked like and felt like – not just the theology of it. Years of ups and downs with my brothers and sisters who have also had their ups and downs. But I too have learned the stability and joy – yes, the anchor – that obedience is for us in turbulent seasons. May God give us all this desire for, and living of, faithful obedience to the life and fellowship he has called us all to in him.

Joann Longton, New London, Connecticut

Thank you for this timely post. I was commissioned by my church to leave England and go to Estonia only last week. Sat in Kiviõli, a town in the Russian enclave, wondering why and what the Lord has for me to do! Our God knows all our needs and all the plans, I first must be still and wait on him.

Nigel Parrott, Kiviõli, Estonia

CARE OF CHILDREN

On the forum "Charting the Future of Pro Life": This idea of having every child born taken care of by the community is a joke. Our Congress won't give an extra dollar for the care of children if they can help it. If you are a single mom making ten or even fifteen dollars an hour, you really can't afford to pay for childcare in a decent center. Where I live in South Carolina childcare alone can run from seven hundred to a thousand or more dollars a month. An apartment can run $875 to $1420 a month and that doesn't include utilities. Add the cost of a car to take a child to a safe space for the child to stay and then the cost of gas and don't forget car insurance. It takes more than a single mom can make. Oh yes, then there is health insurance.

Jacquelyn Weddington,
Greenville, South Carolina

NOT PERFECT

On Dori Moody's "A Broken but Faithful Marriage": I am very touched by this memoir of your grandparents whom I grew up knowing. I saw their struggles and you gave me understanding and compassion for them. It's a fact of life that one can't fix everything even with love and care; some brokenness is too deep, but somehow the message of love, faith, and commitment still shines through.

Leah Maendel, Morris, Manitoba

Such a heartfelt, honest, reflective story. Life is not perfect this side of heaven and yet God is with us, ever kind, loving, good, and just, a rock and anchor for our soul in every storm of life.

Margaret Baird, Belfast, Northern Ireland

REMEMBERING RICH

On Bethel McGrew's "Rich Mullins: Ragamuffin, Celebrity, Disciple": For twenty-one years, Rich, called Richard by his friends, was one of my dearest friends. We had all created a loose community of family friends that endures to this day, twenty-five years after his passing. I just wanted to tell you as someone who knew him well, I have read many articles about him and believe that this captures him

better than anything I've ever read. Thank you so much.

Kathy Sprinkle, Cincinnati, Ohio

POETS IN THIS ISSUE

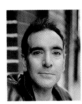

Aaron Poochigian earned a PhD in classics from the University of Minnesota and an MFA in poetry from Columbia University. His thriller in verse, *Mr. Either/Or*, was released by Etruscan Press in the fall of 2017. His latest book, *American Divine*, the winner of the Richard Wilbur Award, came out in 2021. His other poetry collections are *Manhattanite* (Able Muse Press, 2017), winner of the 2016 Able Muse Book Award, and *The Cosmic Purr* (Able Muse Press, 2012). His work has appeared in such publications as *Best American Poetry*, the *Paris Review,* and *Poetry*. His poems appear on pages 49 and 116.

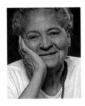

Rhina P. Espaillat was born in the Dominican Republic and came to the United States as a young girl with her family as exiles from dictatorship, settling in New York City. As a bilingual poet, Espaillat is winner of numerous prizes including the T. S. Eliot Prize, the Richard Wilbur Award, and (twice) the Howard Nemerov Sonnet award. *Plough*'s annual poetry award is named for her. Enter submissions at *plough.com/poetryaward*. Her translation of a sonnet by Sor Juana Inés de la Cruz appears on page 111.

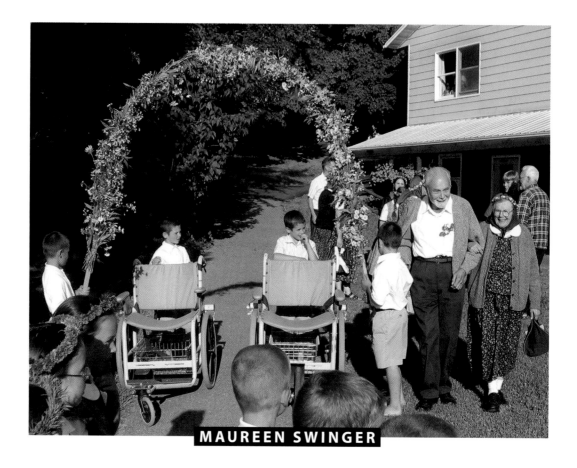

MAUREEN SWINGER

Soldier of Peace

I spoke with the Bruderhof's oldest member,
a World War II veteran, about how to pass on
a spiritual legacy.

PAUL PAPPAS KNEW EXACTLY what he wanted to say to me, and it wasn't going to be about growing old on the Bruderhof (the original topic of the interview), although he'd just turned ninety-eight – the oldest living person in our community movement. He has also been my adopted grandfather for the last twenty-six years, so I was delighted to drive over to our neighboring Bellvale Bruderhof and spend an afternoon catching up. But that didn't mean my questions were getting answered. Not the practical ones, at any rate. To my open-ended "What can you tell me about getting old in community?" he jumped right to the last word:

"Community is the fruit of Pentecost, when the people all of a sudden experienced something so

Paul and Mary Pappas, *right*, on their sixtieth wedding anniversary.

positive that it just brought them together. And we have been brought together in all kinds of ways. Personally, I was very against it to start with, and I have said sometimes that I was too stubborn for God to lead, so he had to close in behind!" He continued, "I feel like when the king wanted to have a big banquet, and he kept trying to get more and more people, and finally he said, go and force them to come in. I was the one who was forced!"

Paul's forceful invitation to community began with his witness to the enormity of war. He had been in the Marine Corps, deployed to the Pacific during World War II. "I landed in Nagasaki six weeks after the bomb was dropped. And I said, 'Why did we have to drop a *second* bomb? Wasn't it clear?'" That gratuitous destruction crushed his faith in almost everything. "When I came out of the military, I was very angry and bitter and cynical. I had no purpose in life. There just didn't seem to be any meaning to it." The one thing he was sure of was that "war was never right. Never. It would never produce what you want, and that is peace."

After the war, his life looked not half bad on the outside, with a young family and career opportunities in electrical engineering. "I was getting to the place where I had a salary and we could have bought a new car, and even think maybe about a house, but I thought, 'What do you do then? You have a new car and you have a house, but so what?' What I didn't realize was that I was missing a purpose, something that I could really do – something to do *about*. As far as I was concerned, religion had no meaning if there was nothing you can do about it right here."

Meanwhile, his wife, Mary, was also searching for meaning and purpose; a talk at a peace conference convinced her that they ought to visit the Bruderhof then in Paraguay. "She said, 'There's something I should do with my life, but I don't

know what it is. When I see it, I'll know it.' And did she know it! She was ready to pack her bags and go. With a baby and a two-year-old.

"She got a vision of God's coming kingdom. It wasn't just community. I'm so thankful for this life. It obviously saved me and it saved my marriage. It was nothing I did." Paul emphasized that he did not share that vision immediately, but credited "God and my wife" for bringing him around. "We have to get the essence of our common life – *why* we're doing this, and the *importance* of it. Because it's for the whole world,

---

"The world was going to hell, and there wasn't anything I could do about it. But now I know what to do about it." *Paul Pappas*

---

not just us. We have been given a task to represent something of God's kingdom here, so that people can see it, can experience it – and that's what had to happen to me. When my wife and I finally went to Woodcrest, I saw something of this. Here was a people who had a purpose, and they were going at it with everything. It dawned on me, well, I don't have that purpose, and I want it. That's what made the big change in me, and it led me, from there on. Because before, I didn't believe people could live like this. No way."

I looked down at my scribbled questions. He was blasting past "Do you feel fulfilled; do you have a purpose for living?" Paul may have took pride in showing up on time in the furniture workshop every day, but that's not what got him up every morning. He made sure to bring the conversation

---

Maureen Swinger is a senior editor at Plough. *She lives at the Fox Hill Bruderhof in Walden, New York, with her husband, Jason, and their three children.*

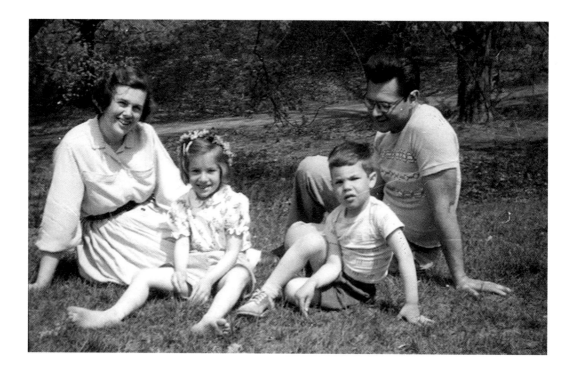

back to that: passing on a legacy, one that was entrusted to his generation, and one that he prayed my generation and the ones following after would fully comprehend. He sympathized with young people's sense that "the world was going to hell, and there wasn't anything you could do about it. But now I know what to do about it." He quoted Eberhard Arnold: "'We have to make God's invisible church visible.' That's our task."

Specifically, he'd been occupied recently with some young men whom he cared for very much. He'd been worried that they'd embraced a sort of simplistic patriotism without wanting to hear that there are dark sides to every power, or that the flag can be an idol. "What I always say is that whatever our country does that's good, it's good – and they do many things that are good. We are very blessed that we are able to live all these years here without being persecuted. We have been accepted, and we have the freedom that we wouldn't have in many other countries. And we have to be very thankful for this. But there are so many things that our country does that aren't right. Even Isaiah says that a time will come when what is said to be good

will be bad, and what is bad is good."

"There are things happening now that in my early years, I would never even have dreamed of," he continued. "We live in a very, very serious time; I don't remember a time in my lifetime when we [as a country] were so divided, and not only divided, but to the point of there being hatred, in so many different things." He worried about signs of war. "Personally, I feel we're in the end times. Just because we live in such a beautiful place – it's peaceful, and we can take care of ourselves, and we can go to work, and everything works out. But that could change overnight."

Paul believed in responding in faith rather than joining the fight. "Sometimes there's a certain urge to get out and protest. I'm not interested in protesting. It doesn't give you a positive answer. But *we* have an answer here. We don't have an army, we don't have a police force, we don't have a justice of the peace; we have to give up something in order to have that. And it's *me*. It's not a question of material things, it's *me*." That kind of self-dedication means becoming part of something greater: "The apostle Paul compares

The Pappases with their two oldest children, 1965.

the church to a body, and if you're baptized, you become part of that body. You're no longer an independent person. You're still yourself, but you act as part of a body. And we find the way together; this is the secret of our life."

I wish the youths who don't agree with him or perhaps avoid his challenges could have heard how invested he was in their future: "One of the guys that I was concerned about – all of a sudden, I don't know what happened, he got up and made a very clear statement; he wanted baptism. I had prayed that somehow God would work in his life. I almost got up and shouted, 'Hallelujah!'"

Once upon a time, *I* was the callow youth Paul and Mary took in: when I was a rather scruffy eighteen-year-old, my first year away from my family, they simply loved me into their household, no matter what I did or said. They listened to my big questions, and were too generous to serve up easy answers. They just had a way of being there, making space for a soul to grow. When I left for college, I knew they were still there for me. When I spent a year working in a migrant center on the edge of the Everglades, I often thought, "What would Paul think about this? What would Mary expect of me?" Their care had power.

When I made my own decision to join the Bruderhof a year or so later, they wrote a letter of celebration and also of vulnerability, telling of the time of their membership vows, and some of the joys and struggles faced in the intervening years. When again, a few years later, we ended up living on the same community, I had a standing invitation to hang out once a week and talk through life. When Mary was dying, I could come and say goodbye and thank her for her love, and she thanked me for being part of the family. I had brought a bouquet of roses from my small garden out back; she exclaimed over each of them separately, rejoicing in practically every petal. That was always Mary's way, and not just with flowers.

When my future husband asked me to marry him, one of the first places I went afterward was Mary's grave. It was a joyous visit; I brought her roses and prayed for a marriage as steadfast as theirs. When Jason and I told Paul about our engagement, he gave us his and Mary's blessing; doubly powerful considering one member was weighing in from heaven. He wrote several thoughtful letters to us as we were just starting out that we still treasure. When after several years

---

Once upon a time, *I* was the callow youth Paul and Mary took in: a rather scruffy eighteen-year-old experiencing my first year away from my family.

---

of marriage we hit tough times, he was solidly in our corner in prayer and quiet counsel, and when we came through, he was first to rejoice with us, with that look on his face that said, "We've been there too."

If Paul were to read this, he would point out that they are not special in any way. They are not the only elderly folk on the Bruderhof who have enough vision to share it around – if we listen while they're here to talk.

Paul's parting words of the afternoon: "We can't be thankful enough for what God has blessed us with. But we are going to be tested, and we need to have our feet on the Rock to face the future. We have to be willing to stand up for what we know is true, regardless of the consequences. If that isn't clear to us, we're not going to make it. How do you pass all that on? I don't know how!"

"Don't give up on us," was all I could think of to say, and he replied, smiling, "Oh no, I have no intention of giving up."

It was our last conversation. Three weeks later, Paul joined Mary in heaven. ➤

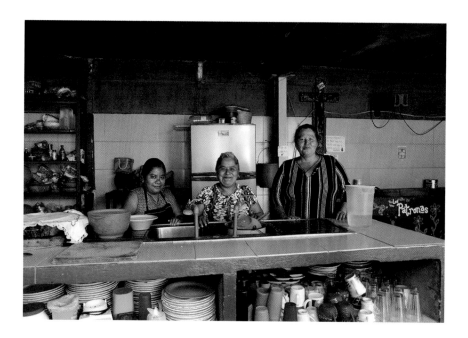

The Faces of Our Sons

*In Guadalupe, Mexico, three generations of women
feed migrants riding the trains north.*

MONICA PELLICCIA

IN TWO HOURS the cargo train called the "Beast" will reach the rural Veracruz town of Guadalupe, in eastern Mexico. Julia, Norma, Bernarda, Teresa, and other volunteers – Las Patronas – begin to cook rice, beans, and eggs with chili. They heat tortillas and fill bags with the food. Some prepare water bottles that will have to be thrown to the people on the cargo train, where hidden migrants make the dangerous journey north, mostly from Honduras, Guatemala, and Nicaragua.

Around 8:30 p.m. a whistle blows, and the women run to the railroad with their boxes of food. But the engineer doesn't even slow down; most of the food bags land on the ground.

THIS IS A DAILY ROUTINE for Las Patronas; not even Covid stopped them in the work they have been doing for almost three decades, since Valentine's Day, 1995. That day a group of Central American migrants shouted from the train to sisters Bernarda and Rosa Romero. "*Madre, tenemos hambre,*" they called. "Mother, we're hungry." The sisters and their mother, Leonilia – they are sugarcane farmers – began to

Julia Ramírez, Maria Teresa Aguilar, and Norma Romero of Las Patronas.

prepare food for migrants fleeing gang violence and poverty, and seeking opportunity or family reconnection in the United States.

"It is a huge satisfaction to help people who need it," says Bernarda. Over the years, she adds, with word-of-mouth reports and media attention, they've expanded their project. "When we started twenty-seven years ago, migrants were not so much in the line of fire of criminal and police extortions," explains Norma Romero, a coordinator. Every day, Las Patronas prepare food bags to give to the migrants on trains and take care of those in their shelter. They treat their wounds, help with bureaucracy, and give them shoes, clothes, and a safe place to regain strength.

"Migration is a business: we are a business," says a Honduran father hosted in the shelter. "The gangs kidnapped us and asked our family for ransom," adds his son, who is helping clean beans in the kitchen. "They covered our eyes, then beat us with a cane for four days. Why is it easy to move for some people in the world but not for us?"

"We saw our sons in the faces of the migrants," remembers Julia, who has been part of Las Patronas for twenty years. "Before I joined, one day, a sixteen-year-old migrant boy entered my patio and asked me for a taco. He had not eaten for three days, and reminded me of my son the same age," she continues through tears. "His eyes were looking at me so deeply."

"That changed everything," she adds. "I decided to dedicate myself totally to the migrants and I came every day. Knowing them helps us to break the narrative that they are criminals."

Keeping going year after year hasn't been an easy task. The women faced criticism from some neighbors: "Why are you helping those criminal people? Why don't you stay at home taking care of your husbands?" some asked them, suggesting that their charity work could land them in jail.

But for all this time they've worked as a mostly female team, trying to overcome stereotypes about migrants and raise support through donations and volunteer help.

OVER THE YEARS, Las Patronas – a play on the town's full name, "Guadalupe (La Patrona)," which in the plural means "female

---

That day a group of Central American migrants shouted from the train. *"Madre, tenemos hambre,"* they called. "Mother, we're hungry."

---

bosses" – involved their families, friends, and neighbors. Patronas like Nancy Mota, twenty-five, and Maria Teresa Aguilar, thirty-eight, are part of the third generation. Both of them have family members who immigrated to the United States. "I see my father in their eyes. He left when I was seven," says Nancy, who joined two years ago.

"I was working as a housekeeper, seeing the train go by every day, with people asking for food. I was wondering to myself: What can I give?" says Teresa while she cooks *chilaquiles*, corn tortillas cut into quarters and lightly fried. "I hope that we can inspire others."

Local support for Las Patronas has grown stronger over time; local donors offer rice and beans, and long-term volunteers help out. Uriel, Alejandra, Edgar, and Itaviany help with tasks from cooking and delivering food to administrative support. And humanitarian donations and support come from farther away as well – donors include the International Committee of the Red Cross.

"I feel the bittersweet impact of this humanitarian work," says Itaviany, while cooking rice

---

Monica Pelliccia is an Italian freelance multimedia journalist who covers environmental and social issues. She has produced reports for Mongabay, the Guardian, El País, *and other international media outlets.*

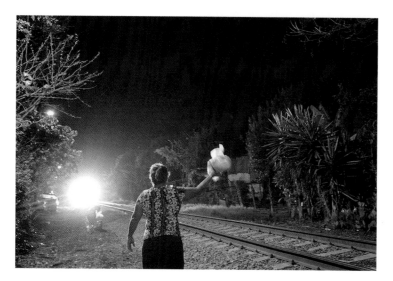

of ten migrant women are raped as they make their way through Mexico. These numbers are drawn from complaints; no one knows how many times it happens to women who are too afraid to report assault, or those who don't know how to.

AS WITNESSES of human rights violations, Las Patronas work without any state support to shed light on migrant stories. In 2013 the group won the Mexican National Human Rights Award; it established a reputation as human rights defenders and members often give talks to universities and schools. "We never expected to share our experience in public," says Julia. "I've lost the fear of talking in public: we always invite people to help migrants and learn their stories. There are so many little things that everyone can do."

The hazards of the migrant trail remain immense: in 2021 the disappearances of Central American migrants in Mexico quadrupled, with more than a hundred thousand people on official lists. This year Las Patronas hosted a group from the Caravan of Central American Mothers, who were traveling the route of the "Beast" in search of their missing sons and daughters.

Las Patronas continue to ask for national policies with greater respect for people's lives and dignity. After the deaths of nearly fifty migrants in a trailer in Texas, during the late June heat wave, they wrote to Mexican president Andrés Manuel López Obrador: "How many migrant lives do we need to lose before national and international institutions can work to bring dignity to people who are migrants?"

"We dream of a change in migration policies," concludes Norma. "We will continue to dedicate our lives to this mission. We invite people to know and help migrants. Any one of us could find herself in their place." ⤳

and beans. "This is the second time I've come; they are like a family to me." It is a feeling shared by other volunteers such as Edgar from Mexico City. "Here," he says, "I learned that doing things without expecting a reward is a way to work toward a better world."

"AFTER TWENTY-SEVEN YEARS, there is still a lack of governmental policies for migrants: they are left alone in the streets and exposed to abuse," says Norma Romero. She is sitting on the kitchen patio, in front of a mural map of Central America. *Los sueños también viajan*, it says: dreams travel too. The mural has portraits of migrants Las Patronas have helped over the years. Some, like Gonzalo and Jaime, reached the United States; others, like Kelvin, died falling from the trains.

Among them, the most vulnerable are the women and girls. "A lot of women decide to cut their hair, bandage their breasts, and inject contraceptives before migrating," writes Alejandra Uribe Aguirre, volunteer and researcher in rural development at Autonomous Mexican University of Xochimilco. "Some of them prefer to make pacts with one person during their journey to offer sex in exchange for protection rather than be raped multiple times by different persons."

Though there is a lack of official data, the Mexican National Commission of Human Rights and Amnesty International estimate that six out

Julia Ramírez awaits the oncoming "Beast" train, holding a bag of food for the driver in the hopes that he will slow down.

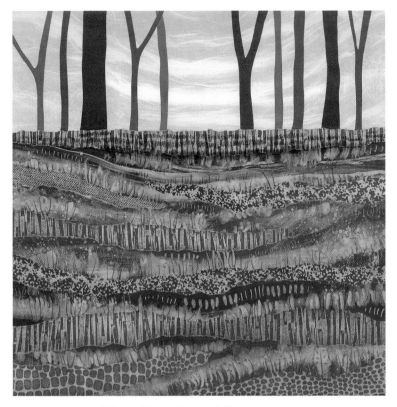

Rebecca Vincent, *Roots and Shoots*, monotype

Yearning for Roots

We're born with a hunger for connection with our ancestors – both biological and spiritual.

PETER MOMMSEN

IN APRIL 1977 the historian Alex Haley arrived in Utah to receive an honorary doctorate in humanities from Brigham Young University. At that moment, Haley's star was rising, no doubt one reason the university was eager to include him in its commencement exercises. Having coauthored Malcolm X's autobiography twelve years earlier, now his bestselling book *Roots: The Saga of an American Family* had just won a special Pulitzer award. A TV miniseries based on the book, which recounts Haley's family history back through slavery to his African forebear Kunta Kinte, had proved a ratings sensation; 85 percent of US households had tuned in to the finale three months earlier. Haley's work sparked an upsurge of interest in family history among

Americans of all ethnic backgrounds, including African Americans, many of whom had assumed till then that their family lines prior to emancipation were untraceable. After Haley, genealogy was no longer just for blue-bloods and *Mayflower* descendants. Family history was democratized.

More lay behind the university's invitation than Haley's celebrity, however. Then as now, the school was affiliated with the Church of Jesus Christ of Latter-day Saints (LDS), commonly known as the Mormons, and so had a specifically theological reason for honoring the author. Mormon religion places a high value on knowing the names of one's ancestors. In the words of its founder, Joseph Smith, "The greatest responsibility in this world that God has laid upon us is to seek after our dead." Unlike traditionally orthodox Christian churches, Mormons see it as an act of filial duty to identify one's ancestors so as to vicariously baptize them into the faith; accordingly, the LDS archive maintains the world's largest genealogical database. These beliefs lay behind the university's justification for offering the honorary degree:

> We see in what Alex Haley has done a remarkable example of the hearts of the fathers reaching down through generations to the children, and the hearts of the children reaching back to their fathers. And if, as Mr. Haley has suggested, "Grandma, Cousin Georgia, and those other. . . . 'up there watchin'," if, as he says, "it was one of those things that God in his infinite wisdom and in his time and way decided should happen," we here, of all people, can understand and honor his great work in responding to these impulses.

Haley's project may have dovetailed neatly with his hosts' genealogical beliefs. Awkwardly, though, his African ancestry did not. At the time, LDS doctrine forbade Black Mormons from baptizing their own ancestors, or for that matter from performing any other of the religion's solemn rites. The reason for this race-based exclusion? Genealogy again, this time in the form

of a doctrine of hereditary taint. Mormonism, following earlier speculations by some Christian, Jewish, and Muslim writers, taught that Black Africans had inherited the "curse of Ham" pronounced by the patriarch Noah on his youngest son's descendants in the Book of Genesis. (By contrast, most biblical scholars believe the passage refers to the ancient Israelites' enemies, the Canaanites.) It was only in 1978 that Mormon leaders would rescind the ban.

No doubt to his hosts' relief, Haley didn't take public issue with the LDS's racial theology when he came to Utah, instead praising its advocacy for genealogical research. "Families need to get their history recorded," he told a reporter for the LDS newspaper *Deseret News*. "Talk to the oldest members of the family about the most minute details they can recall. Once they are gone, they are irreplaceable." Family history, he said, could help address "the pervasive rootlessness that afflicts America."

Haley's diagnosis still applies forty-five years later. Even with the easy availability of information online, many are astonishingly ignorant of even their most recent forebears. One 2022 study found that only 47 percent of Americans could name all their grandparents, while only 4 percent could name all their great-grandparents.

This might seem surprising, since the past two decades have seen a rise in the popularity of new family history services that combine traditional genealogy with DNA testing (sometimes offering genetic health reports as well). Two in ten Americans say they've taken a DNA ancestry test, while over a quarter say that a close relative has. It's a lucrative industry: the pioneering firm 23andMe went public in 2021 with a valuation of $3.5 billion, while the current market leader Ancestry, founded by two Brigham Young graduates, sold in 2020 for $4.7 billion and reports continued growth.

Yet the success of family history services is less

a sign of a robust connection to past generations than of its absence. That's most obviously the case for adoptees or for children born as a result of gamete donation, who may turn to DNA tests to find out more about their biological ancestry. But for other users too, such services by their nature will be most revealing for those who know the least about their family tree beforehand. If you never did get around to recording the memories of your oldest family members and making their stories your own, at least you can get a report on your mitochondrial haplogroup or a pie chart showing your percentage of Nigerian, Norwegian, or Neanderthal genes. That may be sufficient if all you want is proof that you're Irish enough to drink on Saint Patrick's Day. But by itself, genetic data accomplishes little in the way of linking you to the individual human beings who are your forefathers and foremothers.

THE "PERVASIVE ROOTLESSNESS" that Haley identified afflicts not only America, but also virtually everywhere that modernity has touched. Whatever occasional interest people may take in their family history is too weak to overcome a far stronger current of indifference bordering on hostility toward the past. In the words of the Belgian critic Paul de Man, "Modernity exists in the form of a desire to wipe out whatever came earlier, in the hope of reaching at last a point that could be called a true present, a point of origin that marks a new departure." If all that matters is the now – what philosophers call *presentism* – then there seems to be little we can learn from past generations. Instead, the cult of youth wields near-total cultural power.

One result is that the old are cut off from the young, socially and often physically as well. Traditionally, the role of elders was to pass on inherited wisdom to the next generation. But if the past is judged useless or morally suspect, the elderly can seem to have little to offer their communities. Even China, a country proud of its Confucian

tradition of filial piety, felt compelled in 2015 to pass an Elderly Rights Law requiring grown children to visit their aging parents.

This bitter truth is now coming home to the once-young-but-now-aging radicals of the Age of Aquarius. And the wheel keeps on turning. Since the turn of the millennium, the pace of techno-

> **Traditionally, the role of elders was to pass on inherited wisdom to the next generation. But if the past is judged useless or morally suspect, the elderly can seem to have little to offer their communities.**

logical churn has accelerated the expiry date of youth for each generation. The same Millennials who wield the "OK Boomer" meme against sixty-somethings find themselves mocked by Zoomers for their skinny jeans, avocado eating, and cringe emoji use.

The devaluing of the old was laid bare during the Covid-19 pandemic, with particularly high mortality among those living in nursing homes, who also tend to report higher rates of loneliness and isolation. According to a study published in the *Journal of Health Economics,* in 2020 residents of US nursing homes were twenty-three times more likely to die of Covid than Americans age sixty-five and older with different living arrangements; in at least five states, one-eighth of nursing home residents at the beginning of that year were dead by its end.

The sheer number of deaths is a crass illustration of what Pope Francis calls "throw away culture," in which the old, rather than passing on their wisdom to the young, are warehoused until

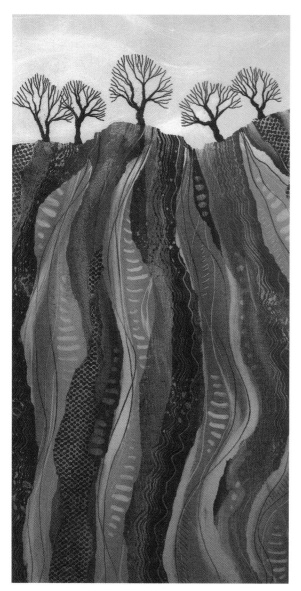

Rebecca Vincent, *Hidden Depths*, monotype

begin to see themselves this way: with no cultural script of reverence for the wisdom of age and respect for its honor, the aged believe themselves to be above all in the way.

It's not only the elderly who are negatively affected when the links between generations break down; the young lose out too. When the hollowing-out of intergenerational connections deprives youth of the sense of belonging to a story beyond themselves, other sources of identity will fill the void. As often as not, that will mean affiliating with an online tribe, which offers a sense of belonging that may range from trivial to noxious. Either way, it's an unstable and risky way to form one's identity.

IN THE COURSE of writing this, I decided to take Haley's advice and look up my own family history. I wasn't interested in paying a tech firm for the privilege of giving it my (and my family's) DNA information. But thanks to Mormonism's continuing commitment to genealogy, the LDS archive now makes records available free online as FamilySearch, offering a handy tool so users can quickly assemble their own family trees using its vast database. Within ten minutes of registering on the site, I found the names, marriage details, and birth and death dates of forebears for each of my grandparents reaching back centuries – it turns out I'm a mongrel mix hailing from Surrey, Wales, Zurich, Ulster, and the Baltic.

Many of the names in the most recent generations were well known from family stories I heard growing up. Certainly my grandparents and great-grandparents are people to whom I feel a genuine connection and sense of duty. These are the people, after all, whose visions, struggles, and sacrifices made my own and my children's existence possible. What's more, these ancestors often live on in their descendants, glimpsed in inherited personality traits, quirky interests, or the familiar profile of a face. In their case, the florid wording

they die. In Francis's words: "The elderly are so often discarded with an attitude of abandonment, which is actually real and hidden euthanasia! It is the result of a throw away culture which is so harmful to our world." Meanwhile, literal euthanasia, in the form of "medical assistance in dying" (MAiD) now legal in several jurisdictions in North America and Europe, is also becoming increasingly common as a logical extension of the same way of thinking. Most insidiously, elders of Brigham Young University's commendation of Alex Haley makes a sort of sense when it speaks of the "hearts of the fathers reaching down through generations to the children, and the hearts of the children reaching back to their fathers."

But go a few generations farther back on the family tree, and it is populated only by strangers – ancestors who, in all probability, I and my kids share with tens of thousands of others, so that to speak of a family relationship seems meaningless. Modern genetics, in fact, suggests that blood relationships at this distance may rapidly become illegible from one's DNA. Or to illustrate the point another way: anyone of European descent is statistically guaranteed to be biologically descended from Charlemagne (likely there are parallel figures for other population groups). Was Haley's quest for identity through researching family history mistaken all along?

An answer is suggested by the genealogies in the Bible. As Alastair Roberts writes elsewhere in this issue, one of scripture's most unmodern aspects is its penchant for long recitals of begats, from Genesis to the New Testament. The genealogies at the beginning of the Gospels of Luke and Matthew, for example, establish Jesus' identity as the "seed of David," tracing his descent back through the Judean kings to the patriarchs, Noah, and Adam. By an odd coincidence, Matthew's version groups the genealogy into sets of fourteen generations – the outer limit, according to today's geneticists, for tracing a specific trait back to an individual ancestor.

But of course, this particular genealogy is precisely *not* a record of the flow of DNA. Genetically speaking the Davidic bloodline stops with "Joseph the husband of Mary, of whom Jesus was born, who is called Christ." As Matthew is about to recount in the following chapter, Joseph is not Jesus' biological father.

Over the centuries, interpreters have labored to explain how Jesus is the "seed of David" if the genealogy of his adoptive father is not actually his.

(Augustine, for one, argued that Mary as well as Joseph was biologically descended from David, and so Jesus belonged by blood to the royal line after all.) But for Matthew, the question of biological descent seems to be secondary. His purpose in beginning his book with a genealogy is not to track the transmission of genes, but to tell the grand intergenerational story into which Jesus was born: the story of God's covenant with his people Israel, of sin and exile, and of the promise of redemption.

Matthew's genealogy, then, both affirms the significance of family history and powerfully relativizes it. Biological kinship, it turns out, is far less important than the family called into being by God's promises. In this sense, Matthew's table of begats is of a piece with an anecdote he reports eleven chapters farther along. "Who is my mother, and who are my brothers?" Jesus asks a crowd of listeners, then answers: "Whoever does the will of my Father in heaven is my brother, and sister, and mother."

In Christian teaching, this redefined family is known by another name: the *communio sanctorum,* the fellowship of saints. In this great intergenerational family, we are linked by a bond of brotherhood and sisterhood to believers from every era of the human story, past, present, and yet to be born. To be sure, our biological families and inheritances still matter; the New Testament pointedly echoes the Decalogue's command to honor father and mother. But heredity and blood kinship are no longer the primary source of our identity. In a prophecy that Christian tradition interprets as describing the age to come, the Book of Zechariah promises that the generations will one day be bound together once more:

> Thus saith the Lord of hosts; There shall yet old men and old women dwell in the streets of Jerusalem, and every man with his staff in his hand for very age. And the streets of the city shall be full of boys and girls playing in the streets thereof.

If there's a cure for rootlessness, it is here. ➤

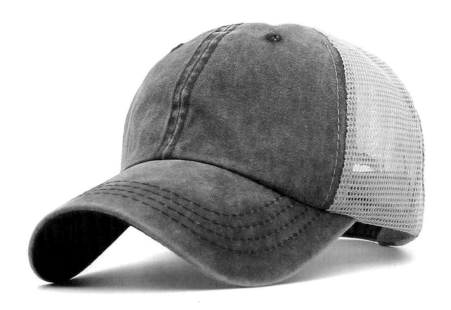

My Father Left Me
Paperclip

*What kind of inheritance can an
illegitimate son expect?*

TERENCE SWEENEY

I HAVE IT ON MY DESK right now. I tied a yellow ribbon around it. Not for any symbolic reason, just to make sure I don't lose it or mix it up with the other paperclips on my desk. I first learned of this inheritance on a train platform in West Philly after getting off the Market-Frankford Line and waiting for the Norristown train. I was on the way to teach. My mother called to say, "Your father died." His lawyers had reached out to her because they needed to contact his surviving children. Since I am still alive – along with my siblings – the lawyers needed to contact me about the paperclip (although I didn't know about the paperclip yet and neither did they).

We spoke briefly. I asked how she was feeling. She said she wasn't surprised; he was older; she just hoped her children got what they deserved (definitely not thinking of the paperclip). I asked about his name again. I couldn't remember, and checking my own last name doesn't help. My mother's maiden name is my last name, which makes my passwords both less secure (if you know my name, you know her name) and more secure (wouldn't Sweeney be the last name you'd pick?). When people ask about my mother's maiden name, I feel awkward. Once as a child I lied and told someone she happened to have the same last name as my father but they weren't cousins. Or I would tell people she wanted to keep her last name and pass it down to us. There is some truth to that.

We got off the phone. I cried, but not because he was dead. I had never met the guy. How do you cry for an absence? For something that isn't there,

a gap in the fabric of a family. I cried because there was nothing to cry about. I should have been weeping for other reasons, but I had no other reasons. I boarded the train with people looking at me askance. I went and tearlessly taught my classes. You can't skip class for a man you have never met.

AFTER THAT, THERE WAS not much news. I called my brother and sister. I talked with my mother, who insisted again that I deserved an inheritance. I looked him up and it did seem that he had been well off: a bank executive with enough clout to serve on the board of a university. My wife and I, who are not so well off, talked about whether I wanted an inheritance. Getting some money would help an artist (her) and a philosopher (me). With an inheritance, we could afford one of the houses in West Philly with a nice porch and tulips. We could have one of those big bay

> I cried, but not because he was dead. I had never met the guy . . . I cried because there was nothing to cry about.

Terence Sweeney holds the Barry Fellowship at the University of Pennsylvania and is theologian-in-residence at the Collegium Institute for Catholic Thought and Culture. He holds a doctorate in philosophy from Villanova University, where he is an adjunct professor.

windows and put a lawn sign up about how we believe in science and that love is love.

At the same time, it would feel weird getting money from a stranger. What would one inherit from a void? He didn't know me, and an inheritance didn't seem like something you would leave to a kid you don't know or, worse, to a kid you vaguely recall as your bastard. A not very charming word. Microsoft Word warns me that this language may be offensive to you, my reader. So I really have no excuse. But it is the right word; it is my word. To be a bastard is to be a person without a birthright and with only half of a family background. Ask me about my paternal uncles or my grandfather on my father's side and I have nothing. A blank on the family tree. I could do some sleuthing, but the fact that I would have to do so is, well, sad. There is no received legacy to pass down. There is no inheritance.

A MONTH WENT BY and then the first letter arrived in the mail. It was a simple legal notice from a law firm on Long Island. They wanted me to verify my address so they could send me further material in the mail. The first letter let me know to wait for the second letter in the mail. I waited.

While I waited, I wondered what would arrive. Perhaps, amid the legal documents, a letter or a photo. I felt the hairs on my neck tingle like I had as a kid on long walks to the lake. Back then, I was sure that the car slowing down would be his. He would hop out and ask me where the Sweeneys lived. For some reason, he was driving with a baseball glove on. Imprudently, I would tell him the way. Returning home, I would find his car in the driveway and casually introduce myself as one of those Sweeneys. He would toss me a glove and suddenly we were having a catch in the yard between the lilac bushes and the broken-down Volkswagen Rabbit. Miraculously, I could catch and throw! He mussed my hair and then headed out.

When the legal package arrived, there was no letter. Just like back then, I found myself at home and still bad at baseball.

The package consisted of a thick manila envelope containing three clusters of paper, each stapled together. Having determined that there was no letter from him to me, I went through the materials. There was in fact a lot of money properly doled out to the "issue of his marriage to ___." The expression came up on page after page, just in case the question was unclear. I was not to receive the inheritance designated for his legitimate *issue*, the half-siblings I had never met. The only place I was mentioned by name was in another packet indicating how I could seek legal recourse for, well, being the wrong kind of issue. When drawing up his will, the man had not forgotten me. A man I couldn't remember and so couldn't forget had remembered me well enough to write me out of his inheritance.

I WAS REMINDED OF THIS at Mass recently listening to Saint Paul: "if children, then heirs" (Rom. 8:14–17). But some of us are children and not heirs. Some of us had a father without ever having a dad. Yet here Paul is speaking of a deeper sonship, one that includes even us bastards:

All who are led by the Spirit of God are children of God. . . . When we cry, "Abba! Father!" it is that very Spirit bearing witness with our spirit that we are children of God, and if children, then heirs, heirs of God and joint heirs with Christ.

I felt that as a child. I found real solace as a kid saying the Our Father. It wasn't the same as saying "my dad," but the universal compensated for the lack of the intimate. Fatherless, I still got to have a Father.

Christianity is a religion for the illegitimate. As Rev. Will Campbell puts it, "We're all bastards, but God loves us anyway." None of us are children of God in any legitimate sense; we are made legitimate by adoption. What's more, we're grafted onto a family centered on a man who was born to a not-yet-wed mother and didn't get to spend too much of his time on earth with his (real) Father. We may get disinherited in this life, but we're adopted by the Father no matter what our status.

As a boy, it was a solace to be able to pray to Our Father and know that even if he couldn't play catch with me, he would stick around. With my own father dead, this prayer gives a bit of solace and connection even now. From the obituaries I learned that Catholicism is something I shared with my father. When I prayed the Our Father, I now know, he too may well have been praying the Our Father. A tenuous connection but more real than any in my fatherless youth.

I SET THE PACKET DOWN on my desk and heard the light tap of metal on wood. A stack of legal documents held together by a paperclip. Nothing to hold on to, nothing to pass on. I took the paperclip off and dropped the will in the trashcan. I held the clip in my hand. A paperclip, well cared for, could last a long time. My father had paid the law office for the work, the documentation, and all the material that went into making sure I did not receive anything. The paperclip was

an ironic consolation; he had left me something after all. I was to receive no inheritance, but my father left me a paperclip. Not much, but not nothing. I showed my wife; she held my hand. I tied a yellow ribbon around the clip and slipped it into my desk drawer.

Where my father had been there was only absence, a space that was barely there. In the rich tapestry of love that my family had woven around me, he punctured a whole. My whole life I had kept vigil for when he would step into a space that I had kept open. He died and left that space as empty as ever. I did not get money from his dying, but I got a reminder: I pray to a Father who has promised, through his Son, to never disinherit any of his children. Perhaps, because of this Father's mercy, I'll meet my father someday. Maybe he'll teach me to play baseball. But in the meantime, I still need something to hold on to from the dad I never had. I have tried to live with absence my whole life, but you can't live with absence. I have always needed something to hold on to. I have my paperclip now; I can live with that. ✒

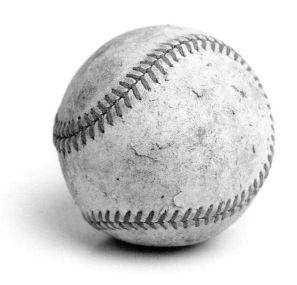

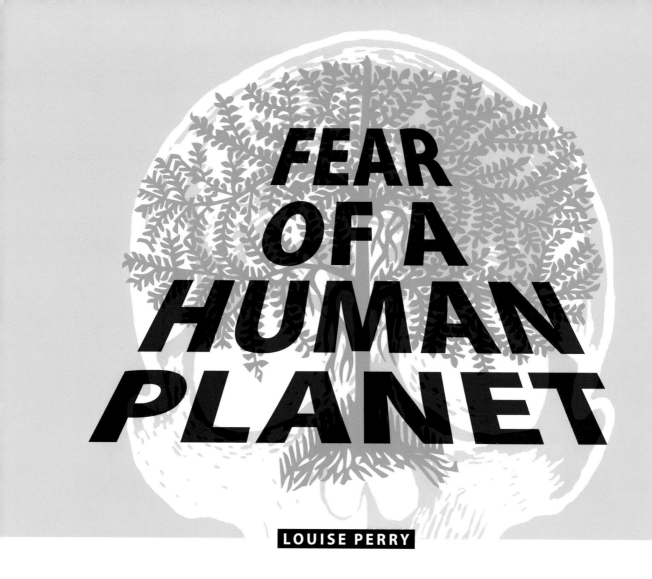

FEAR OF A HUMAN PLANET

LOUISE PERRY

Do children endanger the environment?

GOD PROMISED ABRAHAM that he would make his descendants "as numerous as the stars in the sky and as the sand on the seashore." We must assume that the readers of the Hebrew Bible took this to be a good thing – the greatest of blessings, in fact.

But Lloyd Williamson, an environmentalist activist from Essex, United Kingdom, takes a very different view of his possible progeny.

When he reached his early twenties, as he told the *Guardian*, he thought "You know what? I don't want to bring a life into this world, because it's pretty shitty as it is and it's only going to get worse." At the age of thirty, Williamson underwent a vasectomy. He is among a growing number of people who say they are committing to remain childless in response to the threat posed by climate change.

Louise Perry is a writer and campaigner based in London. She is a columnist at the New Statesman *and a features writer for the* Daily Mail. *Her debut book* The Case against the Sexual Revolution *was published in 2022 (Polity).*

Illustrations assembled from graphics made available on the Extinction Rebellion website.

In a paper published in the *Lancet* last year, among ten thousand people aged sixteen to twenty-five surveyed in ten countries, 39 percent of respondents reported that they were "hesitant to have children" because of climate change. Other surveys find high levels of anxiety among children. One conducted by the BBC in 2020 found that 20 percent of children aged eight to sixteen reported having had at least one nightmare about climate change. Many in this generation are profoundly gloomy about the future of the planet.

Many climate-change campaigning organizations agree with this assessment, and agree also with the goals of "BirthStrikers," environmental activists who have elected to remain childless. Population Matters, for instance, is a UK-based charity that campaigns on global population size and its effect on environmental sustainability. "One of the most effective ways that we can help our planet today is by choosing to have a smaller family," the Population Matters website informs visitors.

With or without the interventions of activists, though, population growth is already waning worldwide. "Demographic transition" is a sociological term that refers to the historical shift from the high birth and death rates that were once ubiquitous across the world toward longer lives and fewer children. The first countries to experience the demographic transition were European, beginning in the nineteenth century, and it has now occurred everywhere, with the exception of some parts of sub-Saharan Africa.

In the 1980s, two Dutch sociologists advanced a provocative hypothesis: that many societies might be undergoing a "second demographic transition" that would lead to birthrates so low they would fall below replacement level. At the time, they were dismissed by their peers, but now their hypothesis has been vindicated. The world population is still growing, but only because of high birthrates in Africa – a temporary reprieve. In almost every other part of the world, the population is shrinking. A paper published in 2020 in the *Lancet* predicted that the world's population is set to peak at 9.73 billion in 2064, and then decline.

Experts are divided on exactly what is causing the second demographic transition. Brad Wilcox, a fellow at the Institute for Family Studies, describes a complex interplay of factors:

> There is an economic story behind falling fertility in the developed world, but there is a cultural story here as well. People who are more religious and conservative seem to have more of a motivation to have kids, and also less fear, including climate fear, whereas people on the left and secularists are more worried about having babies.

Wilcox points out that, while their climate fear is certainly sincere, it is not the only factor at play for those reluctant to have children. There is what sociologists term an "elective affinity" between environmentalism and other lifestyle factors that are known to lead to lower fertility: in particular, lack of religious faith. There is a very strong negative relationship between secularism and fertility, both for societies and for individuals. It seems that people who don't believe also tend to have fewer babies. Looking at data covering more than fifty countries and more than eighty thousand people, sociologist Landon Schnabel of Cornell University found that across many countries, secular people have fewer children than religious people. The effect holds true for societies as well: in more secular countries, even religious people tend to have fewer children than their co-religionists in less secular countries, though they tend to have more than their secular compatriots. Social mores are powerful – but faith can, it seems, push back against them.

Such studies suggest that there is an important spiritual component to the crisis in which we find ourselves. To be sure, there is a real environmental problem that urgently deserves our attention and action. Yet there is also a problem of faith, and it is expressed most clearly in the divisions within the environmentalist movement.

The writer and futurist Alex Steffen describes three categories of environmentalist: "light greens," who encourage lifestyle changes at the individual level; "dark greens," who believe that environmental destruction is an inevitable consequence of industrialized capitalism and therefore work towards radical political change; and "bright greens," who see an answer in technological innovation.

It is the dark greens and the bright greens who are most at odds over the issue of population reduction. From one angle, the dispute is an empirical one: Could new technology plausibly have a large enough impact to avert climate catastrophe? The American economist Eli Dourado is among those who believe it could. "The writing is on the wall," he tells me:

> By the time the decade is out, the majority of cars being sold are going to be electric. Almost-zero-carbon transport is on the way. . . . New

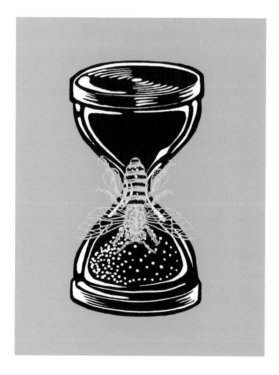

technologies are coming online, like geothermal, which is likely to be very big in about ten years or so. The potential there is enormous: not just lower cost, and lower emissions, but a greater abundance of energy than ever before.

Techno-optimists like Dourado understand climate change to be a technical problem, readily solvable with enough investment. This could come from governments, or it could come from private companies: the billionaire entrepreneur Elon Musk is currently running a competition to find the most effective solutions for pulling carbon dioxide directly from the atmosphere or oceans and sequestering it durably and sustainably. The winner will be awarded $100 million, the largest incentive prize in history. Musk – who has nine children – is resolutely against the "BirthStrike" movement, telling the audience at a *Wall Street Journal* event in December 2021 that "if people don't have more children, civilization is going to crumble, mark my words."

Light greens vary in their sensibilities, but tend toward a less technologically bombastic approach. They often advocate change driven by personal choice – to cycle rather than drive, to take up various "green" practices. Some light greens seek society-wide commitments to live less wastefully, to live with natural systems rather than seeking to overcome them; they sometimes see in Musk-style technology its own temptation toward excess.

Other environmentalists are skeptical of the idea that technological innovation, personal choice, or renewed cultural interest in and commitment to sustainable agriculture alone will avert climate catastrophe. Anna Hughes is the director of Flight Free, a British organization that campaigns to inform people of the climate impact of aviation and inspire them to travel by other means. She has also personally resolved not to have children – a decision she reached in her early twenties, partly in recognition of the environmental impact of population growth. I ask Hughes for her view of the "bright green" environmentalist project:

> Sure, we can try to technologize our way out of this, but we cannot just keep adding to our number because, regardless of how much we reduce our emissions, if we keep on growing then our emissions will keep going up: it's simple maths. So we have to talk about the population question.

To some degree, the disagreement between Dourado and Hughes is simply on the question of timescale. Dourado is expecting the technology to come on in leaps and bounds, and soon – by the end of this decade, say – whereas Hughes is more pessimistic.

But there is also something more temperamental at play in the differences between the bright and light and dark greens. There is a fundamental gap between how these groups of people regard the future, and it is expressed most clearly in their outlook on children – the people who, of course, literally embody the future.

One of Anna Hughes's fellow campaigners told her recently that she felt distress, not so much at the prospect of her children suffering in a world affected by climate chaos, but at the prospect of their loss of faith in the future, that "they will live knowing that all hope is lost."

Contrast this perspective with Elon Musk's project to build human settlements on Mars, a project that Eli Dourado supports, telling me "I think it would be a shame if, within the next century, we are not expanding into the solar system." Faced with exactly the same environmental problem, some people have resolved not to bring any more human life into the world, while others are looking to the heavens and imagining new human lives "as numerous as the stars in the sky." This is in part, again, a question of timescale: Can we get off the earth soon enough? But it is a spiritual one as well.

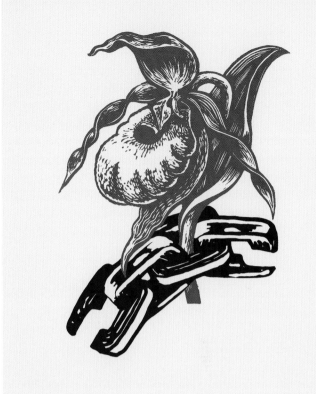

This division of sensibility within various branches of the environmental movement is echoed, though not perfectly, in divisions among political and religious groups. Modern secular progressives – the group least motivated to reproduce, according to Nitzan Peri-Rotem's 2016 study "Religion and Fertility in Western Europe" – have a fraught relationship with both the past and the future. Theirs is a restless ideology that both predicts and insists upon constant renewal in the form of "progress," with new frontiers constantly presented to adherents. We live in a society that is unhappy with its past – really, in truth, unhappy with itself.

Climate change presents a problem for progressive ideology, which comes from a tradition predicated on the expectation of inexorable improvement. But at the same time, progressives are more likely to believe that we will find ourselves collectively faced with catastrophe at some point in the near future. A 2017 study of Americans revealed that around 70 percent of

Democrats believe that major climate-related catastrophes will occur within the next fifty years, while only about 20 percent of Republicans do. Anecdotally, I've found that those who believe in a very definite full stop within our lifetimes due to climate apocalypse are almost always progressive and secular.

"If you're younger than sixty," claimed novelist Jonathan Franzen in a 2019 *New Yorker* article, "you have a good chance of witnessing the radical

---

Modern secular progressives – the group least motivated to reproduce, according to recent studies – have a fraught relationship with both the past and the future.

---

destabilization of life on earth. . . . If you're under thirty, you're all but guaranteed to witness it."

Franzen is also noted for his rejection of those authors in whose tradition he writes, for their regressive sensibilities. "Read a book from fifty years ago by John Updike, Norman Mailer, Thomas Pynchon, Kurt Vonnegut and, even though I love him, Joseph Heller, and you see they weren't thinking about women in the right way," said Franzen in a 2021 interview defending, essentially, cancel culture. "I wish people would be spontaneously sensitive, but if they can't, then a little bit of enforcement doesn't seem to me a bad thing."

Thus progressives like Franzen find themselves precariously poised in the present moment. Both the past and the future are rejected: the former for its sinfulness, the latter for its fearsomeness.

In 1968, *The Population Bomb*, a book written by Stanford University professor Paul R. Ehrlich and his wife, Anne Ehrlich, predicted catastrophe as a consequence of uncontrolled population growth, with hundreds of millions of people set to starve to death in famines that would occur during the 1970s and 1980s. The book was written in a tumultuous year, both politically and culturally, and it evidently hit a nerve, going on to sell millions of copies, aided by the apocalyptic public pronouncements of its author. "Sometime in the next fifteen years, the end will come," Paul Ehrlich told CBS News in 1970. "And by 'the end' I mean an utter breakdown of the capacity of the planet to support humanity."

The Population Bomb's dire predictions did not come to pass, either after fifteen years or fifty and counting. The world's population has more than doubled since the publication of the book, and yet deaths from famine have declined radically since the book was published, from fifty people per one hundred thousand annually during the 1960s to less than one person per hundred thousand anually in the 2010s. As well, world hunger is now dramatically reduced: at the time the Ehrliches wrote, one person in three was chronically hungry; that proportion has fallen to one in nine. This improvement is due in large part to the "green revolution" of high-yield crop varieties that increased food production. In this instance, the techno-optimists were vindicated.

That does not, of course, necessarily mean that they will be vindicated again. But the mistakes of *The Population Bomb* reveal something important about how a febrile historical moment can lend itself to widespread panic about the future. At times of conflict and uncertainty, faith often falters. It's little wonder that one-third of a generation is reluctant to participate in the transhistorical project that is family formation – a project that demands that we place our faith in the future, delivering to it our most precious offering. But though this reluctance is understandable, it is ultimately not sustainable. The future belongs to those who hope. ⤴

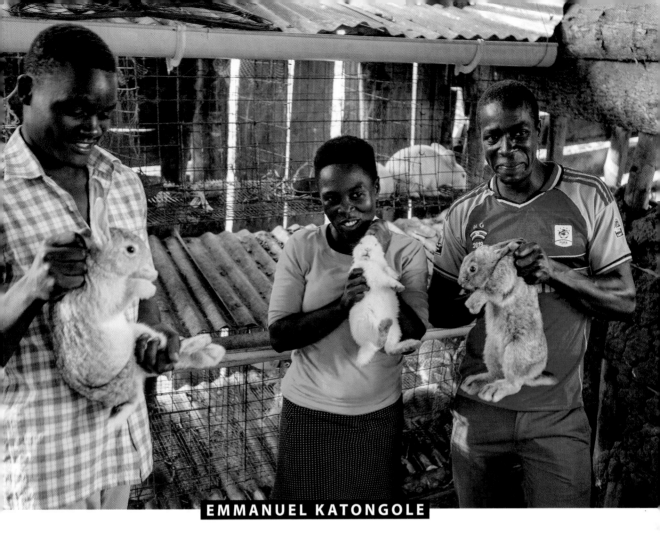

EMMANUEL KATONGOLE

Reviving the Village

*By returning to the land, African Christians seek to
heal the ravages of ecological and ethnic violence.*

DURING THE GENOCIDE in Rwanda in 1994 I was a graduate student in Belgium. We had just watched the BBC evening news with images of dead bodies in streets, churches, and rivers and were leaving the common room in stunned silence when a colleague turned to me and blurted out, "Why do you Africans always kill your own people?"

While grossly unfair and insensitive – I was born to Rwandan refugees in Uganda – this question has followed me through almost three decades of peacemaking and studying two issues at the heart of the question. First, the issue of identity: What does it means to be African? And second: Why is violence so prevalent on the African continent?

Trainees raise rabbits at the Bethany Land Institute's model farm in Uganda.

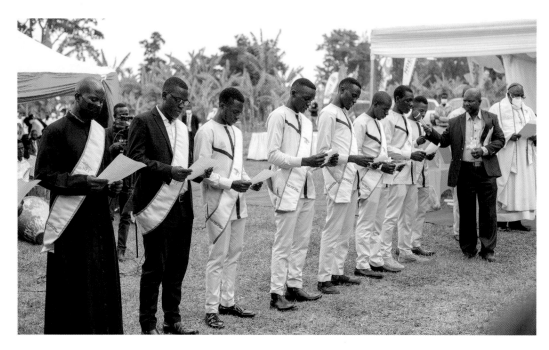

The first cohort of sixteen trainees is officially commissioned in early 2021.

Examining the intersection between identity and violence in Africa has led me to see that the 1994 Rwanda genocide is not separable from but deeply connected to other forms of violence in Africa – ethnic, religious, and ecological. Many people associate violence in Africa with a primitive "tribal" outlook, but this is not the case. There is something distinctly modern about all these forms of violence. Even what usually passes under the label of ethnic violence is a recent phenomenon that reflects unsettled questions of belonging and of who has access to the social, political, economic, and cultural institutions of modern Africa.

Ethnic, religious, and ecological violence in Africa does not constitute three separate forms of violence, but modalities – a better word might be "echoes" – of this ongoing crisis of belonging. One can trace this crisis to a story, first told by European colonialists, in which Africa is at once rejected – "Nothing good can come out of Africa" – and projected as the beneficiary of the European project of civilization, pacification, and development. This story lives on and continues to shape the social, political, and economic institutions of modern Africa, resulting in the image – and thus reality – of Africa as a perpetually disabled, deficient, and violent continent.

Can Christianity offer resources with which to navigate this uniquely modern crisis of belonging in nonviolent ways? Or will Christianity simply amplify it, as often seems to be the case? For Christianity to be helpful, it will need to tell a different story, one that fosters new forms of community that defy static notions of identity, engendering new economic and ecological possibilities in modern Africa.

After all, Christianity is, in its essence, a story: the story of God's love manifested in Jesus' self-sacrificing love on the cross, ushering in for his followers a new identity, a new community, a new people that expands to incorporate all people, and a new social order infused with love. In my latest book, *Who Are My People?*, I tell stories of

Christian activists and communities in Africa whose examples confirm that this is not some utopian dream or merely spiritual idea; it is a concrete social reality today. In the end, it is the antidote to Africa's violent modernity.

Three Faces of Africa's Ecological Crisis

The village, the slum, and deforestation are three interrelated faces of the ecological crisis in Africa. Though over 65 percent of Africa's population live in rural communities, there is a growing impoverishment of life in rural Africa, with increasing water poverty, food insecurity, and lack of viable economic possibilities. Most villages have no paved roads, electricity, health care, or other basic social services. The late Tanzanian president Julius Nyerere once said that while the rest of the world is trying to reach the moon, in Africa we have yet to reach the village. He was speaking not only of the difficulties of physically getting to the village, but of a mindset that ignores the village as irrelevant to development. Still today, in the minds of many government and international development agencies, the village represents what it represented for the colonialists: an image of all that is backward and primitive, all that should be left behind in order to realize the dreams of modernity and civilization.

According to this mindset, the city represents the promises and dreams of civilized modernity. It is therefore not surprising that, lured by dreams of progress, employment, and better living conditions, millions of people, especially the young, decide to migrate to the cities. And while cities in Africa are growing fast, its slums are exploding at a terrifying rate. The 2016 World Economic Forum on Africa predicted that Africa's population of 1.1 billion will double by 2050, with more than 80 percent of that population living in cities and the majority living in slums ("informal settlements") where poverty and violent crime are widespread and basic public utilities such as clean water, reliable electricity, and law enforcement are absent.

Rapid deforestation is another face of Africa's growing ecological crisis. According to the UN Food and Agriculture Organization, old-growth forests in Africa are being cut down at a rate of more than 4 million hectares per year, twice the world's deforestation average. For example, in Uganda forest cover diminished from around

> Ethnic, religious, and ecological violence in Africa do not constitute three separate forms of violence. They are echoes of the same ongoing crisis of belonging.

10.8 million hectares in 1900 to 4.9 million in 1990 to only 1.9 million in 2015. A number of factors contribute to this depletion of Africa's forests – population growth, commercial logging, agricultural expansion, and the use of firewood as a predominant source of energy.

These three faces of Africa's ecological crisis – the burgeoning slum and the vanishing village and forest – confirm a number of things. First, they are evidence of the extent to which the cry of the earth and the cry of the poor are interconnected, as Pope Francis expresses it in *Laudato si'*. In fact, they reveal the unique modernity underway in Africa, characterized by what journalist Christian Parenti has called a "catastrophic convergence" of poverty, violence, and ecological degradation. As Pope Francis notes, addressing this triple challenge requires an

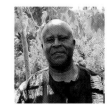

Father Emmanuel Katongole, PhD, is a core faculty member of the Kroc Institute for International Peace Studies at the University of Notre Dame. His latest book is Who Are My People? *(Notre Dame, 2022), from which this article is adapted.*

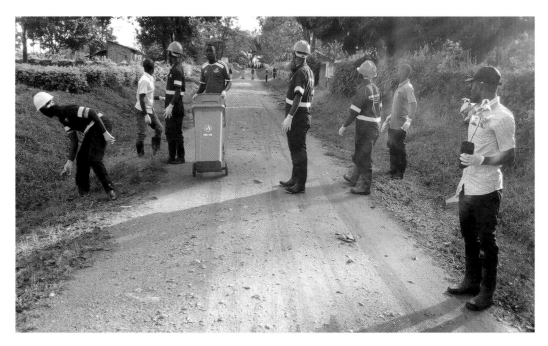

Bethany Land Institute students take part in community service in the surrounding villages.

integrated approach that addresses poverty, cares for creation, and advances human dignity for poor and marginalized people.

Second, they represent forms of what Princeton professor Rob Nixon calls "slow violence." These gradually unfolding calamities remain largely imperceptible, undetected, and untreated. Incidents like flooding and mudslides are just symptoms of the underlying violence. To refer to climate change and ecological degradation as "slow violence" is not simply to say that they lead to violent outcomes (destruction of lives and property) or that they trigger violence (conflicts over diminishing land and water resources), which they obviously do. It is to recognize them, as Kevin J. O'Brien writes in *The Violence of Climate Change*, "as the product of a destructive system that degrades human lives, other species, and the world upon which all living beings depend."

Third, they point to a shifting relationship with nature in general, and land in particular. Perhaps the most obvious evidence of this shift is the rapid rate of deforestation and the destruction of natural ecosystems, but no less important is the rural-to-urban exodus that leads to the growth of slums and the abandonment of villages. Africans' changing relationship to the land is the result of a modern outlook that eschews the traditional spiritualities which encouraged an intimate, symbiotic, and sacred relationship to the earth, which was considered "mother." Modern people view these spiritualities as backward and primitive, and see nature primarily as a resource. Development economics encourages this world-view with its focus on a "cash economy" and its exploitative and extractive relation to the land.

As I've said, underlying this modern outlook is a crisis of belonging, which Acholi poet Okot p'Bitek captures well in his classic set of poems entitled *Song of Lawino, Song of Ocol*. *Song of Lawino* is a bitter complaint – a lamentation by Lawino about her educated husband, Ocol, who has not only left her but abandoned the traditional ways of his people, whom he now looks down

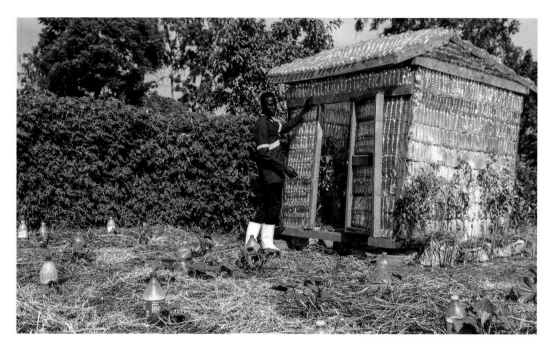

This greenhouse was created by reusing old plastic bottles.

upon as primitive and pagan. He abuses all things Acholi and considers all the ways of his people backward. Lawino appeals to her husband to "return home" and learn to respect the traditions of her people, whose roots "reach deep in the soil."

Ocol will have none of that. For him, the way forward is not to return home but to "smash" the primitive customs and embrace the dreams of progress and civilization represented by the city:

> . . . I see the great gate
> Of the City flung open,
> I see men and women
> Walking in . . .
> Why don't you walk in with the others?

In the end, however, Ocol offers Lawino no choice:

> You have only two alternatives my sister
> Either you come in through the City Gate
> Or take the rope and hang yourself.

It is this total dismissal of tradition and the village – and the acceptance of a Western idea of progress – that shapes the dreams and aspirations of modern Africa. It is enshrined in a particular model of economic development. As economist Jeffrey Sachs notes in *The End of Poverty,* the "ladder of economic development" involves a "progression of development that moves from subsistence agriculture toward light manufacturing and urbanization, and on to high-tech services." This is the dream of economic development promoted by the World Bank, IMF, and other development agencies and embraced by African leaders. What is increasingly obvious, however, is that this vision of inevitable progress, of climbing up a ladder of economic develop-ment, is leaving a huge ecological footprint of deforestation, pollution, mass poverty, and mass unemployment in much of sub-Saharan Africa.

Demonstration Plots for a Different Future

What would it take to redirect this modernity? What would a new economic vision – an "integral ecology," as Pope Francis describes it, one that fights poverty, protects nature, and restores human dignity – look like in Africa? Pope Francis points to the need for "spiritual conversion," and Lawino appeals to Ocol to "return home" to rediscover the wisdom of "our people" whose roots reach deep into the soil. Are there any experiments in this spirituality of deep connection and belonging to the land that could testify to the possibility of a new modernity in Africa? The Songhai Center in Benin and the Bethany Land Institute in Uganda are two such models.

In 1985 Godfrey Nzamujo, a Dominican priest, founded the Songhai Center in Porto-Novo, Benin, West Africa, to address the challenges of poverty, food insecurity, and unemployment in rural communities. To date the Songhai Center has trained over two thousand young people in sustainable and organic farming, value-chain practices, and business-creation skills. More than half these students have gone on to create sustainable farms in their own villages.

What makes Songhai Center an effective answer to the catastrophic convergence of development economics, poverty, and environmental degradation in Africa? Nzamujo identifies three elements at the heart of his efforts.

First, a clear diagnosis of modern Africa's challenges. The story of Songhai Center goes back to the 1983–85 famine in Ethiopia that led to the deaths of over four hundred thousand people. At that time Nzamujo, who had earned doctorate degrees in electronics, microbiology, and development science, was a research professor at the University of California, Irvine. As he watched images of emaciated African children on TV, he felt shame and anger. The images were reinforcing the standard image of Africa as a "hopeless" continent of bloody wars, famine, and poverty, and of its people as helpless victims extending their hands begging for a handout. Africa need not be like that, Nzamujo protested. In his mind was the memory of the great civilizations in Africa's history, like the West African empire of

Songhai in the fifteenth century, which attracted scientists, scholars, students, and merchants from far and near, and built cities like Timbuktu, a prestigious center of learning. What went wrong, Nzamujo wondered, to bring Africans to the point where they seem unable even to feed themselves?

Africa's problem, he surmises, is the "trap of poverty," an "incapacity to effectively harness the opportunities before us." While empires like Songhai confirm that this capacity was available in Africa's past, we have largely lost it and "succumbed to the logic of poverty." Africa's problems of unemployment, poverty, famine, and environmental degradation are all manifestations of this faulty modern logic. Underlying the trap of poverty, Nzamujo notes, is an internalized belief that nothing good comes out of Africa. Accordingly, we respond to Africa's needs using Western solutions and models. This leads to a slavish mimicry of Western habits of superficial consumption. Shaped by a colonial heritage, we perpetuate forms of development economics that primarily benefit less than ten percent of the population. The result of these modern policies, Nzamujo tells me, has been the "erosion of dignity" and the destruction of "Africa's internal capacities to meet the challenges before her."

Secondly, the need for a new imagination. What is needed, according to Nzamujo, is "a new way of looking at ourselves, the world, and others" and "another way of placing ourselves in the world." This will require a paradigm shift, with "Africa learning to harness her internal capacities and local knowledge." While the idea of a paradigm shift might sound heady, for Nzamujo it is a simple thing that begins with, and happens through, working with the land and changing the way we grow food. "God has given us everything we need right here." Working the land will not only stem the problem of rural-urban exodus, it "will recreate the villages as viable social economic units," and thus help in the creation of a new African society. This possibility of

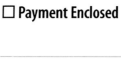
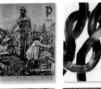

☐ **Payment Enclosed**   ☐ **Bill Me**

NAME
_____

ADDRESS
_____

CITY _____ STATE _____ ZIP _____

EMAIL (FOR E-NEWSLETTER AND UPDATES)

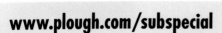

www.plough.com/subspecial

||||| |||

BUSINESS REPLY MAIL
FIRST-CLASS MAIL   PERMIT NO. 65   BIG SANDY, TX

POSTAGE WILL BE PAID BY ADDRESSEE

PLOUGH PUBLISHING
PO BOX 8542
BIG SANDY TX 75755-9769

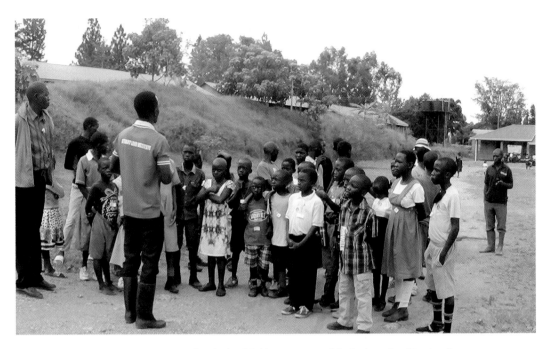

Paul, a trainee, leads a group of local schoolchildren in a tour of the Bethany Land Institute's campus.

reinventing African economics from the ground up led Nzamujo to resign his position at the University of California and return to rural Africa to work on the land.

At the heart of Songhai Center is what Nzamujo describes as a simple logic – namely, that everything is connected. The Songhai model is an integrated system of crops, livestock, and aquaculture, where waste from one unit becomes food for another. This is the primary production, supported by the secondary production of technology, processing, and manufacturing, and the tertiary level of services, such as market, restaurant, and lodging. Nzamujo hopes this microeconomy can be replicated throughout Africa, turning villages, which modernity has coded "hopeless," into viable economic and social units.

Thirdly, a spirituality underlies Nzamujo's work at Songhai Center. This spirituality is an invitation not to fight nature but to work with her. Nzamujo understands his work with the land at Songhai as

"a form of contemplation, and a prayer, which is but a way of entering into the mystery of reality." He refers to Songhai as a "sermon" because "all we are trying to do is to contemplate the dance of nature" and to "imitate the way nature works." Nzamujo sees great affinity between his being a Dominican and his scientific background, in particular his appreciation of quantum physics. The latter, unlike the Newtonian physics of external forces acting on matter, is about discovering the interconnected nature of reality. Accordingly, at Songhai there is no dichotomy between nature and science, between faith and practice, between creation care and scientific production, or between agriculture and techno-logical innovation. Scientific innovation, far from being an attempt to "subdue" or "tame" nature, is just another dimension of the invitation to "enter into the dance of nature" and an example of harnessing the interconnectedness within nature to advance the flourishing of both the human community and of nature herself.

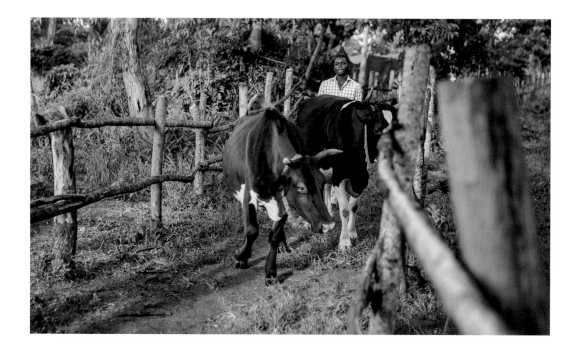

Entering the dance of nature reveals another crucial reality: that human beings are an integral part of the universe and not masters who stand apart from it. Birth leads to death and decay leads to renewal, just as light leads to darkness and darkness leads to light. The more we become connected with the earth, the more we discover that just like the rest of creation, we are part of this cycle of death and resurrection. This became personal for Nzamujo after his own cancer diagnosis. He writes, "If we let go and accept suffering and embrace our death, then we are released. We become fully alive, as we become reconnected to the earth's fragile fertility. . . . The power of the resurrection can only be accessed from our freedom to die. The experience of our fragility or our limitedness becomes a pathway to a fuller life."

P'Bitek's Lawino appealed to her educated husband to "return home" and rediscover the ways of his people, whose roots "go deep into the soil." This is what Nzamujo has done. But his return is not to a pristine subsistence mode of living on – and off – the land. Rather, it is a return to a sense of belonging to the earth. We see at Songhai a new synthesis that overcomes the usual misleading either/or binaries: either tradition or modernity, backwardness or progress, village or city, spirituality or technology, nature or science, past or future. What we see at Songhai is the invention of a new modernity, one that is not built on the rejection of Africa but whose roots go deep, both literally and metaphorically, into African soil. This soil is in itself a mystery, within which one also discovers that everything is connected. The integration of science and technology with the skills of crop, animal, and fish farming reflects and enhances this interconnectedness.

Inspired by what I witnessed at Songhai, and later also by Pope Francis's *Laudato si'*, I decided to return to Uganda from my post at Notre Dame University to help establish Bethany Land Institute, another center that seeks to cultivate this vision of integral ecology among young people in rural communities. With two other Ugandan Catholic priests, Cornelius Ssempala and Anthony Rweza, I acquired ninety-five acres in Luwero, Uganda, site of some of the bloodiest clashes in Uganda's long civil war. In the Bible, Bethany is a place of refuge where Jesus often returned to teach, rest, and find comfort among friends. We named our institute after this place and our programs after Jesus' three friends there: Mary's Teaching Farm, Martha's Market, and Lazarus' Forest.

In 2021 we welcomed the first cohort of sixteen students, called Caretakers, into an intensive two-year residential program to learn practices of regenerative agriculture, reforestation, and entrepreneurship that they can then take back to their villages. The Caretakers commit to training four apprentices on their own farms in the following two years, and to freely sharing their knowledge with everyone. In this way, the Caretakers will become an ever-expanding network of knowledgeable, caring, creative farmers.

A New People and a New We

I've focused here on ecological violence. A similar analysis of Africa's ethnic and religious violence reveals the same underlying crisis of belonging, which reflects the persistence of a colonial imagination in the so-called postcolonial age. Here too, what we need is a new mindset, a new outlook, a new imagination. Christian identity, it seems, could offer such a new way of looking at ourselves and others, of "placing ourselves in the world," as Godfrey Nzamujo puts it. But since life in Christ is an undeserved gift, it is a way of being placed by God in the world. Christian identity, however, is not static. Our placement in the world is an invitation to constantly cross boundaries into an ever-expanding sense of "my people." This is a "new we" that moves beyond the boundaries of race, nation, ethnicity, gender, or tribe.

Here one can rightly speak of Christian spirituality as politics. The late Archbishop of Bukavu, Emmanuel Kataliko, invokes this politics of spirituality, and its apparently contradictory logic of "simplicity" and "excess," when in 2000, at the height of war in the Congo, he writes a pastoral letter from exile to the Christians in Bukavu. In it, he reminds the beleaguered Christians that "the logic of the gospel is a logic not of power but of the cross." In the end, this simple message is the Christian response to the violence in Africa. For, as Kataliko reminds the Christians, "the only response to the excess of evil is the excess of love."

Amid the recurring and widespread suffering and wanton sacrificing of African lives, Nzamujo and other Christian activists I have interviewed across the continent have come to see their own suffering within a bigger drama: the story of God's own self-sacrificing love. This means that healing the wounds of Africa's violence will involve another form of violence, which Óscar Romero has called "the violence of love." For these men and women, God's love not only allows them to embrace the reality of their suffering, it "heals," "liberates," and "releases" them from fear, unleashing a new freedom. Out of this newfound freedom, they are able to "invent" new communities and practices through which they seek to heal, restore, and renew other victims of violence. Through these "inventions" one is able to grasp the possibility of a radical transformation of Africa's suffering: from the sacrificing of Africa to the true sacrifice (*sacra facere* is to make sacred) of Africa, from sacrificing others to self-sacrificing service, from a love of violence to the violence of love.

There may be no good answer to that terrible question posed to me back in 1994: "Why do you Africans always kill your own people?" But I hope that in the midst of the madness of ongoing violence, places like Songhai and Bethany Land Institute can help us see evidence of another future emerging in Africa.

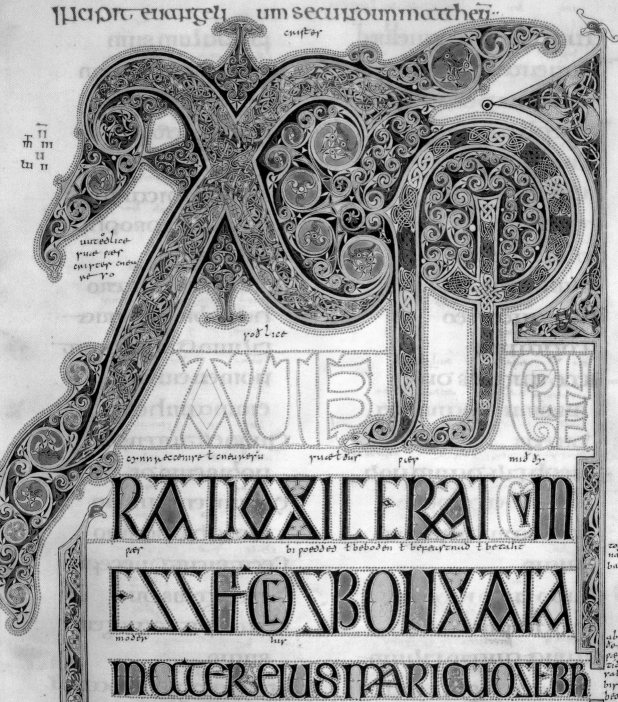

onginned   godppell   efτ
ILICIPIT euangeli   um secundum matheu
                                              cuipter

th   ıı
th   ıı
     ıı
lu   ıı

uutedlice
piuet pap
cuıpeap enou
ne po

poþlıce

cynnpeccenıpe t eneunepıu   puet dur   pıep   mıd þy

per   bı poedeþ t beboden t bepeupnud t betælıt   togemar
                                                                          nallep t
                                                                          banne.

RATIOXILERATCM

ESSHOSBONXA

moden   lup   abıacha
                                                                       de aldom
                                                                       pep ınd
                                                                       tıd ın hı
                                                                       palem p
                                                                       byıcob lıt
                                                                       beoþ ma
                                                                       ıop eph
                                                                       gemenn
                                                                       tobeggeop
                                                                       annıt m
                                                                       claenm

moττeReusmariaⱳoseBR

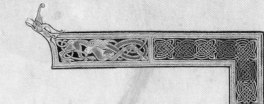

Decoding the Bible's Begats

We moderns tend to think genealogy shouldn't matter. Scripture disagrees.

ALASTAIR ROBERTS

EVERY FEW YEARS, dozens of members of my wife's extended clan descend upon a small cabin next to a lake near Mystic, Connecticut for a reunion. Newcomers to the family are initiated into its culture, a sediment of peculiar traditions and customs that have accumulated for the better part of a century. As it was the first reunion since I married into the family, Susannah and I had to perform a ceremonial leap into the lake from the pier. I was given a tour of the trees on the property that memorialize deceased members of its former generations. She also sewed a leaf-shaped piece of fabric representing me onto the larger hanging of the family tree.

Susannah and I belong to Gen Four of the extended family tree; the family has now attained to its fifth generation. The members of this most recent generation – and the news of expected additions – represent the promise of continuation and the family's shared life into the future. As Neil Postman once observed, "Children are the living messages we send to a time we will not see."

Participating in such an event, I was recalled to the importance of the ways that the meaning of our lives transcends their brevity. We are bearers of the legacies, memories, and hopes of those who preceded us, custodians who must hand them on to others, hopefully in a form enriched by our temporary possession. The meaning of our present labors and sacrifices

The Lindisfarne Gospels manuscript, from which the artwork in this article is taken, dates back to ca. AD 700. Historians believe that Eadfrith, a monk at Lindisfarne, an island off the Northumberland coast, was both scribe and artist of the manuscript. The image opposite, from the Gospel of Matthew, shows the first letters of Christ's name.

is entrusted in part to descendants we may never even meet, much as we represent a harvest rewarding those of our ancestors.

The New Testament begins in a surprising manner. If one were to ask most people to rank different forms of biblical material according to how interesting they are, one would not be culmination. The gospel narrative does not begin in a historical vacuum, but as the climax of a long history of God's dealings with Abraham and his descendants. Matthew's catalog recalls familiar names that represent some of the narrative's most important moments, recollecting earlier events and characters so that the hearer recaptures the

---

The gospel does not begin in a historical vacuum, but as the climax of a long history of God's dealings with Abraham and his descendants.

---

surprised to find genealogies taking up the bottom slots, along with such things as instructions for sacrificial rituals and lists of offerings from the book of Numbers. Yet Matthew chose to open his Gospel with the pyrotechnics of a genealogy. In the prominence he accords it, Matthew recalls the Old Testament book of the Chronicles, which begins with nine chapters of genealogies, upon whose rocks lie the wreckage of many a well-intentioned Bible-reading project! Indeed, Chronicles appears to be one of the sources that Matthew has drawn upon. To the curious contemporary reader, the prominence enjoyed by Matthew's genealogy invites close attention and reflective consideration.

An important and pervasive feature of biblical literature is intertextuality – texts regularly echo, recall, allude to, cite, and otherwise play off each other. As a result, much of their richness cannot be properly appreciated unless we read them in conversation with various others. Matthew's genealogy is no exception.

A genealogy such as Matthew's is a way of alluding to and evoking a larger narrative, not unlike the "previously on . . ." recap before the first episode of a new season of a television series. It situates new events within the arc of a larger narrative, of which they will serve as the

threads of the greater story. This, of course, is one of its most important purposes: any who might otherwise be tempted to regard the New Testament as entirely self-contained are immediately charged to understand Matthew's account against the vast backdrop of the Old Testament.

To many readers, Matthew's opening "the book of the genealogy . . ." (Βίβλος γενέσεως) would immediately have recalled the repeated formula of Genesis, the same words used in the Greek Septuagint. In his purposeful echo of this familiar and prominent expression, Matthew evokes this background: Genesis is the great book of beginnings and the gospel is the account of a new beginning in the middle of history.

As Peter Leithart has recognized, the Gospel of Matthew employs the entire scope of the Old Testament narrative as a template. What better way to communicate the way that Jesus bears, contains, and fulfills the destiny of the people of God than by recounting his ministry in a way that constantly evokes the memory of the older one? With his allusion to the generational formula of Genesis and the character of Abraham, Matthew begins as he means to go on.

The story of Genesis will be even more powerfully evoked: another Joseph bar Jacob is given

---

Alastair Roberts received his PhD from Durham University, and teaches for both the Theopolis Institute and the Davenant Institute. He participates in the Mere Fidelity and Theopolis podcasts. He and his wife, Plough *editor Susannah Black Roberts, split their time between New York City and the United Kingdom.*

prophetic dreams and leads his family down into Egypt for safety. Here there is another king killing baby boys, from whom the child appointed to be the future savior of his people is again delivered. However, in a twist on Exodus, the king is in Israel and the refuge in Egypt. Later, Jesus spends forty days in the wilderness being tested, as Israel was tested for forty years.

Such biblical patterns continue to play out in the Gospel, which climaxes in the death and resurrection of Christ, framed to allude to the destruction of the temple and the exile of Judah, followed by the rebuilding of the temple and return from the far country in the resurrection. Fittingly, its final verses – the Great Commission – echo the concluding verses of 2 Chronicles, in some orderings the final book of the Old Testament.

Apart from Jesus Christ, two key figures stand out in Matthew's genealogy: Abraham, with whom it begins, and David, arguably its pivotal figure. Abraham was the father of the Jewish people, called from Ur of the Chaldees, who received the promise that his descendants would be numerous as the stars of heaven. David was the great king, the founder of the ruling dynasty, the one from whom the promised Messiah was to arise. Jesus is introduced to us in the first verse of the Gospel as "the son of David, the son of Abraham." These titles are far from incidental: he is introduced to us as the bearer of the great burden of expectation and destiny.

The genealogy itself contains forty-two generations, ordered into three movements: "So all the generations from Abraham to David were fourteen generations, and from David to the deportation to Babylon fourteen generations, and from the deportation to Babylon to the Christ fourteen generations." The genealogy is not comprehensive: it omits three wicked kings between Joram and Uzziah. The 14-14-14 pattern

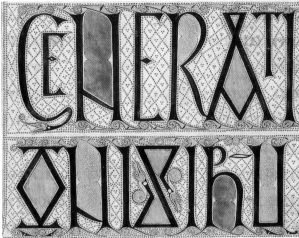

is likely an intentional literary design, inviting comparisons with the cycles of the moon, as James Bejon has argued: there is a period of waxing from Abraham to David, followed by a period of waning from David to the exile, and another period of waxing as Israel is raised up from its exile, culminating in the arrival of the Messiah.

The number fourteen, as several commentators have noted, also has a particular association with David, the climax of the first group: it's the gematrial value of his name in Hebrew. The second fourteen ends with the collapse of the Davidic dynasty in the descent into exile. The final fourteen ends with the advent of the Davidic Messiah, framing the story of David's throne and Jesus as David's true heir.

While Matthew's genealogy generally proceeds from father to son, prior to the introduction of Mary four women break up this pattern: Tamar (verse 3), Rahab (verse 5), Ruth (verse 5), and Bathsheba ("the wife of Uriah" in verse 6). Were we to pick out notable women from Jesus' line, these probably would not be the first to come to mind! The great matriarchs – Sarah, Rebekah, and Leah – are nowhere mentioned, yet women with more complicated histories are. Tamar, likely a Canaanite woman, became the mother of Judah's children through an act of deception, dressing as a prostitute in Genesis 38. Rahab, the Canaanite prostitute who harbored the spies in Joshua 2 and was delivered from the fall of Jericho, is nowhere else mentioned in association with Salmon, yet here we are told that she married the son of the prince of the tribe of Judah (1 Chron. 2:10–11). Ruth was a Moabite widow who married Boaz, a descendant of Lot's incestuous relations with his daughter (Gen. 19:37). Bathsheba was the wife of the Gentile Uriah, wickedly taken by David, who then engineered the death of her husband.

By mentioning these four women, Matthew primes his hearers for narrative themes that frame both the birth of Jesus and the wider character of his work. The first thing they highlight is the inclusion of Gentiles among the people of God: each of them was a Gentile or, in Bathsheba's case, formerly married to one. If the ancestry of the Messiah includes all these Gentile women, is it not fitting that many Gentiles should be within his bride, the church?

Their stories also describe times where the covenant was in jeopardy, stories of courageous faith, of forgiveness, of life from the dead. In Genesis 38, for instance, we witness the house of Judah descend into death: Two of Judah's sons die, his wife dies, and Judah refuses to give Tamar to his youngest son, Shelah, to continue his line. Only through Tamar's cunning deception does the chapter end with the birth of two sons and, even then, the line of one of them is condemned to frustration. The resourceful Rahab bravely hid the two men who spied out Jericho and was rescued from a condemned city. The loyal Ruth raised up life to a dead man's line and gave her mother-in-law, who had abandoned hope, having lost her husband and two sons to famine, a son in her old age. Bathsheba and David lost their first child through the Lord's judgment: the birth of Solomon was a sign of forgiveness and of life from the dead. Through these women Matthew alludes to a long history of the Lord's bringing in the foreigner, forgiving and restoring his people, and raising up David's line from the clutches of death, as well as the daring faith and love of weak and victimized outsiders who trusted in this salvation. In the resurrection of Jesus, God will raise up David's Seed once more.

We might also consider how these women become mothers in surprising or irregular ways – as with the culminating story of Mary, things are not necessarily as they first appear.

Matthew's recounting of Christ's genealogy is a reminder that the hope of David's line never lay in its own vigor but in the power and promise of the God who can open a virgin's womb and a sealed tomb. Joseph, described in verse 20 as "son of David" himself, will become father to the Messiah, but not from his own strength.

Jesus took upon himself the troubled history of David's line, with all its sins, frustrated hopes, and tragedies, and lived out its destiny restoratively, to fulfill the promises to Abraham, that his line would bring blessing to the nations.

Moderns have become dulled to our own place in the generations, to the ways that we receive, bear, and pass on legacies, to the ways we are the harvest of former generations' labors and how our own labors await the harvest of future generations. In Matthew's genealogy, Jesus is introduced to us through the patterns of a long succession of earlier generations, as the fulfillment of their hopes, and their redemption from tragedy, frustration, and death.

Much of scripture traces God's gradual work of deliverance and restoration over many generations of a people. It reveals the legacies of past sins, but also the remarkable ways that his salvation can restore and reverse them. Implied in the promise to Abraham that all the families of the earth would be blessed (Gen. 12:3) may be not only the hope that all peoples might come under the beneficent rule of Israel's Messiah, but that the overcoming of tragedy and the gift of fulfillment exemplified in David's line, accomplished by the Son of Abraham, might be worked out in our family lines too. ➤

Is There a Right to Have Children?

The fertility industry pushes IVF as an answer to the pain of childlessness. But at what cost?

MATTHEW LEE ANDERSON

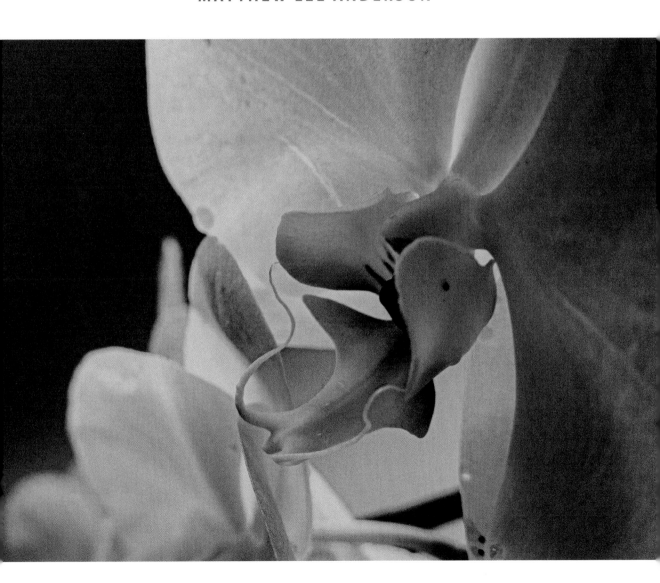

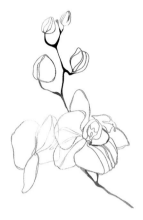

IN THE WANING DAYS of World War II, J. R. R. Tolkien published *The Lay of Aotrou and Itron*, a five-hundred-line medieval-style poem. "No child he had his house to cheer," Tolkien writes of the aging Aotrou, "to fill his courts with laughter clear." Aotrou's anxiety about his "empty pride" and the dissolution of his lineage moves him to seek out a corrigan, a medieval witch, whose fertility potion gives him and Itron the heir they wanted. "Tis sweet at last the heart's desire to meet," Itron happily exclaims, "thus after waiting, after prayer, thus after hope and nigh despair."

The desperation Tolkien depicts is familiar within scripture, and even the use of fertility-enhancing drugs. In Genesis, Rachel so intensely wants a child that she uses a surrogate. Not satisfied with that, she then trades access to Jacob for Leah's mandrakes – the ancient Near East equivalent of fertility supplements. Similar stories abound: Sarah, Rebekah, and the Shunammite woman all faced the devastation of childlessness. And who can forget the tears of Hannah, that patron saint of childless women facing one more Mother's Day at church?

While the prayers of these women to bear a child are ultimately answered, the story of Aotrou and Itron reads like a prophetic warning against taking human creation into our own hands at all costs. Nothing comes free from witches in medieval fairy tales, and Tolkien's modern rendition is no different: the witch demands Aotrou leave Itron, and then takes his life when he will not comply.

In 1978, thirty-three years after Tolkien's story was published, the first baby conceived using in vitro fertilization (IVF) would be born. While contraception was the first wave in reshaping how humans conceive of sex and childbirth, the success of in vitro fertilization was the second. For the first time, technology offered the power to meet our desires for biological children.

Since then, nearly ten million children have been born worldwide through IVF, each of them a blessing for which their parents have no doubt felt inestimable gratitude, each of them a beloved child of God. But the widespread use of IVF technology has come with its costs as well. The first is exacted from the other children created in the process: for every live birth, several other embryos – unique, nascent humans, as we all once were – have been brought into being. Some of these are implanted in the mother but naturally miscarry. Many are discarded in the lab as being of "poor quality." Some are genetically screened for conditions that, by the logic of the screening, make them unworthy of life. Some (fewer than you might imagine, given the heated bioethics debates of twenty years ago) are donated to scientific research. And some – an estimated million in the United States alone – remain indefinitely on ice, their parents unable to decide what to do about them.

There are many other costs to IVF, of which the astonishing price tag is perhaps the least significant. Couples who pursue IVF will bear the

---

Matthew Lee Anderson is an assistant research professor of ethics and theology at Baylor University's Institute for Studies of Religion and the associate director of Baylor in Washington.

burdens of doing so in their bodies: the regiment of hormonal treatments, autoerotic "pleasures" in sterile offices, and extractive surgeries all take their toll. It intensifies an already asymmetrical burden on women, by adding invasive procedures to the process; it imposes unknown risks on children, who are transferred and stored while in an exquisitely vulnerable condition at the origins of their life; in screening and discarding nascent human beings with the "wrong" genetic profile, it perniciously qualifies the value of lives based on their characteristics and reaffirms a conditional attitude toward human dignity that is by no means confined to the IVF laboratory.

But what is all of this against the powerful desire for a child? Against this imperative, few objections survive; as the desire becomes a demand, anything must be done to meet it.

In the United Kingdom, soon after the first IVF baby was born, fertility doctors began to speak of a "right" to have a child. This social transformation has dramatically reconfigured what it means to be infertile.

In recent years, a movement to establish "fertility equality" for nontraditional couples has grown. At bottom, the movement redefines "infertility" as a social fact, rather than a medical reality. Anyone who is unable to conceive, for whatever reason, now counts as "infertile" – including those who are single or in a same-sex relationship. By appealing to the "right to have a child," the fertility-equality movement can justify surrogacy relationships and other nontraditional means of bringing humans into this world. It will likely succeed, given the West's astonishing laxity about procreative norms. The United Kingdom, Canada, France, Israel, and other countries provide state funding for IVF, and were it not for the United States' hopelessly complex healthcare system, it would not be far behind.

At the same time, the success of IVF has meant that other therapeutic interventions are being neglected by the fertility industry. Childless couples today find themselves in a medical environment that hurtles them impatiently toward IVF, which has the joint advantages of both being relatively successful and highly lucrative (though it is not nearly so successful as many people think). Meanwhile, *Fertility and Sterility*, the journal of the American Society for Reproductive Medicine, published a number of essays in 2019 naming the

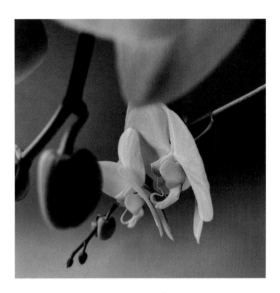

crisis of declining skills and diminishing education for therapeutic interventions and surgeries besides IVF. Couples wrestling with involuntary childlessness who are unwilling to embrace IVF face a medical complex that not only regards their concerns as unintelligible, but increasingly lacks the skill and interest to help them investigate the underlying sources of infertility without skipping straight toward artificial reproductive technologies. The first-line approach to unexplained infertility by many clinics is often intrauterine insemination (IUI). This older procedure does not result in "extra" embryos or genetic screening. Yet it still involves introducing third parties into the process of procreation, creating a formal division between the act of intercourse and the conception of a child. As a result, many Christian ethicists regard IUI as dubious. Either way, the financial incentives and relative success rates of IVF mean many couples are urged to pursue it regardless of whether alternate means might succeed.

It is among the many ironies that the same society that pushes IVF toward the end of child-bearing years does much to discourage having children till that point. While some young people might willfully delay marriage and childbirth, the vast majority have been unintentionally swept along with an economic and social environment that has been built on denying their importance. Meanwhile, declining birth rates around the globe have revived pro-natalist sentiments in the United States and elsewhere. As the sterile world that P. D. James imagined in *Children of Men* becomes more like reality (already, Japan has turned to

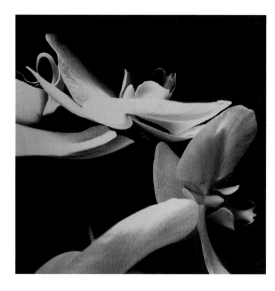

using dolls to simulate the presence of children), a layer of social as well as personal urgency enters the question of whether or how to have a child.

Christians are not immune from these mixed messages. In certain circles, there is a stigma on childless couples who have apparently disobeyed the putative "command" to procreate in Genesis 1:28. For a great many people, the burden of childlessness is a cross not of their own making. Those who prate about how young people are

turning away from children are often the same people who filled those young people with upper-middle-class expectations, and demanded they get the college degrees to meet them, adding physical and financial obstacles to family formation. It is not surprising that a generation of Protestant Christians who had no patience for the celibacy of Jesus in their theology of marriage now have no accounting for the (biological) childlessness of Jesus in their theories of procreation. Meanwhile, many churches have been silent about IVF while our society has trapped a million embryos in ice to await Judgment Day; the Southern Baptist Convention, for example, has said nothing since IVF was introduced.

For Christians, the idea that there is a "right" to children is, theoretically, foreign. We are far more likely to think that children are one of God's good gifts, and that the complex of medicine is simply one new way God has given us to receive them. Yet we are more susceptible to the logic of rights than we realize, even if we do not use the language. When we face the cross of childlessness, we might not invoke our "rights" in our prayers. But we often embody them within our actions. Our claim to children is more felt than articulated – but it is no less real for its tacit expression.

Children are an unmitigated blessing from the Lord. Yet Tolkien's tale is a stark reminder that the gifts of God can be loved in the wrong ways. The consolation childless couples need lies elsewhere, away from the industrialization of fertility and the "rights" it tempts us to claim. How has our vision of children and procreation has been distorted, and how it can be repaired?

Good and Gracious Gifts – Gone Wrong

The tragedy of childlessness is real, and unspeakably deep. Childlessness means gaps in the common life of friendship with other parents, whose all-consuming kid activities are a reminder of what we are missing out on. It means confronting loneliness in old age and wondering who will bury us if we outlive our siblings. More than those, though, it means the absence of a lineage, of descendants who carry on the name we were given and that we forged through our character and life. The one with children stands proud "at the city gates," Psalm 127 says, because children form the reputation of their parents as no one else can. The command to honor parents is tied to living long on the earth, which secures a name for both the parent and the child: in this sense, children are an "inheritance from the Lord" (Ps. 127:3). Begetting a child is an assertion, in deed if not in word, that it is *good* to be our selves, together with the one we love, and that we need not be ashamed of such goodness. To face infertility soberly and honestly is to squarely address the question of the value of our own existence and life.

Theologians have sometimes met these frustrations with blunt appeals to the gospel, which in their reading more or less demands that childless couples *get over it*. Karl Barth offers the glib (even if true) word that childless couples "must set their hope on God and therefore be comforted and cheerful." More recently, theologian Michael Banner's antipathy toward the unmet longing for children prompts him to argue that moral theology should "deny the existence of (and repudiate) the desire for the child of one's own," and "*deny the tragedy of childlessness* which that child is intended to relieve." Unlike Barth's position, Banner's view has the misfortune of being both callous *and* false. The goods of nature are real goods, and we cannot so quickly move past our sorrow for not receiving them.

While the tragedy of childlessness is real, though, it is of a peculiar sort. It is not the tragedy of being denied what we are owed, of not receiving our due. We have no more a "right" to conceive a human being than we have a right to marry one. The way a relationship begins shapes its character, and framing the parent-child relationship through the language of "rights" distorts it from the outset. The nature of parental love is sacrificial: to give gratuitously and to endure the long, joyful, and sad series of goodbyes as the child enters the mature freedom of adulthood. To consider children an entitlement introduces a possessiveness into the relationship that is antithetical to such a love and inimical to both parties' flourishing. Through the deep struggle to set aside these unfulfilled desires and trust the kindness of God, childless couples (paradoxically) learn to cultivate the very form of sacrificial love they long to share.

It is better to think of children as a gift. The paradox of procreating is that it involves so many limits on our agency – that there is so much beyond our control. It is plausible to think that all we can do is *try* to procreate, as the success of any particular act of intercourse in generating life is highly contingent: so much luck and so many inefficiencies are involved in forming human life that one might reasonably doubt the intelligence of the process's designer.

The advent of artificial reproductive technologies might seem to correct this design flaw. But in doing so, IVF suggests that childlessness is a disease. If IVF is a "therapeutic" intervention on par with dialysis machines or other medical treatments, then there is something *wrong* with the couple who has not conceived. Many infertile couples already feel "broken." Medicalizing the creation of a child inherently reinforces that perception, making childlessness even more of a burden than it was before.

Instead, in relinquishing control, a couple may find that the luck and contingencies involved in bringing life into the world also bind them together: to attempt conception requires, after all, the frequent and successive uniting of a couple in love. Theologian William May once wrote that sex must be "intended to be *open to* the gift of life," which is an odd formulation. After all, it is rare to think we *intend* to be *open* to a gift. We generally think we intend what we can bring about ourselves. What child, after all, "intends to be open" to receiving a gift at Christmas? Yet the vulnerability within the process of generating human life puts sharp limits on what we can do in bringing new life into the world. We can be the occasion for God's action in generating a life who bears the image of God – but we cannot compel him to do so.

Such an approach allows for genuine grief when such a gift is not given. The blessing of the Lord precedes, accompanies, and surrounds Genesis 1:28's exhortation to be "fruitful and multiply." Whether command or something else (and I think it is *not* a command), the generativity of a people is a mark of divine favor upon them. It is a fine thing to seek blessings from the hand of God, and an occasion for sorrow when we are not given them. Yet that grief is intrinsically qualified by the limits on our agency, and the claims we can make in light of them: because we cannot bring about a child, we must release ourselves into the hand of God.

Childlessness is not a pathology in need of a remedy, but rather a disclosure of the deepest truth about human life: that it comes from God. In the unfulfilled desire for children, couples come face-to-face with the fundamental core of human existence, the sheer givenness of our life behind which we simply cannot go and for which we must simply be grateful – that we live and move and have our being only as the gift of God. Such is the cross and calling of childless couples.

The Household and the Cross

Every Christian couple who uses IVF has their reasons. Finding the grief of infertility intolerable and the hope of IVF irresistible is more than understandable. It takes either masochism or heroic strength to oppose the temptations to satisfy the longing for children by making life within the laboratory. These parents are as much victims of the lordless powers as willing participants in their

regime. In a world where getting what you want remains the only principle, it seems especially unjust to tell the childless that they must live with unfulfilled desires. No one else is, after all.

If we look beyond the industrialization of fertility, though, we will find that we are *all* implicated in the impulse to escape the limits of our flesh of which artificial reproduction is only the outer edge. This issue merely makes the refusal to honor our bodies more transparent.

Western society's widespread desensitization to the body has made it increasingly indifferent toward other, more violent forms of manipulating nature. What began with efforts to help infertile couples has culminated in the wildly unregulated use of surrogates, an exploitative practice that threatens to sever the link between birth and parenthood. Stranger forms of making life lie on the horizon, too, as in vitro gametogenesis will enable us to make human beings out of stem cells from any combination of humans, and artificial wombs promise to free women from the burden of gestation altogether. This seamless, anti-life garment of "control" extends to the end of life as well: we increasingly pursue medical treatment to the uttermost in order to forestall death, on the one hand, while turning toward the euphemistically named "medical aid in dying" on the other. The reshaping of our society's imagination on matters of life and death seems to know no limits.

The first step to forming Christian imaginations in the realm of sex and marriage is to expand their horizons in a different direction. The gospel offers an account of the human family that is less simple and more inclusive than the odes to the blessing of procreation may suggest.

Even the Old Testament qualifies the value of a biological lineage in palpable and sometimes shocking ways. Hannah's song after birthing and releasing Samuel not only offers hope to the childless but issues judgment on those with children: "The barren has borne seven, but she who has many children is forlorn" (1 Sam. 2:5). That song is echoed in Psalm 113:9: God "gives the barren woman a home, making her the joyous mother of children." "Sing, O barren one, who did not bear," the Lord says in Isaiah 54:1, "Break forth into singing and cry aloud, you who have not been in labor! For the children of the desolate one will be more than the children of her who is married."

The desolation of childlessness has its home on the cross, and its hope in the resurrection. The childlessness of Jesus remains the great qualifier and challenge to any pro-natalism, as his life opens up the possibility of a kinship that transcends (without destroying) the value of procreative bonds. While Mary is the biological mother of Jesus, Joseph (who some sources suggest was an adopted son himself) willingly takes the role of his

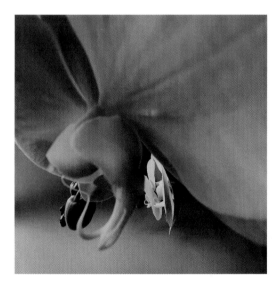

earthly father. Then, on the cross, Christ reconfigures his household by giving his disciple John filial responsibilities to Mary and offering Mary maternal privileges over John. These endorsements of "fictive kinship" pervade the Gospels.

The vision of the New Testament must be embodied, though, through the retrieval of the Christian *household*. To speak of the household means looking beyond the "nuclear family" – a stunted, insular vision that limits the dimensions of family life and our solidarity with others outside our homes. As a "place of mutual and timely belonging," in Brent Waters's words, the household is a gathering place for a wide variety of social relationships in which the joys of marriage radiate outward in a form that is adverbial – through *parental* relations, rather than *parenthood*. And it is a place where care and support can be given in ways not bounded by biology, but by the responsibilities we accrue to one another within the providential care of God's kindness. Whoever does the will of God is Christ's mother and brother and sister (Mark 3:35). In the same manner, we may be father and child and uncle to all those whom God calls us to love.

No book has modeled this vision so well as C. S. Lewis's *That Hideous Strength*, in which the Director's house at St. Anne's on the Hill becomes a refuge for the intentionally childless Jane and the involuntarily childless Dimbles. Jane's troubled marriage and determination to not have a child – "One had one's own life to live," she thinks to herself – collide with the Dimbles' generous love, which is parental without being smothering, and which bears fruit for the kingdom through their obedience.

While Cecil Dimble had been Jane's tutor before her marriage, Mrs. Dimble "had been a kind of universal aunt to all the girls of her year." Their house had been a type of salon, yet of all Dr. Dimble's students, his wife had felt for Jane "that kind of affection which a humorous, easy natured and childless woman sometimes feels for a girl whom she thinks pretty and slightly absurd." Mrs. Dimble feels the sorrow at the empty rooms in her house, yet embodies maternal virtues toward Jane all the same. The childless Dimbles had the luxury of a ready supply of young people to regularly fill their home, which not all couples do. Yet they embody the expansiveness of love that is necessary to overcome our tacit or explicit demands to meet our "right" to have a child. Indeed, the whole household at St. Anne's is a picture of the fruitfulness of chastity – in marriage that is open to children, whether or not God gives them, and

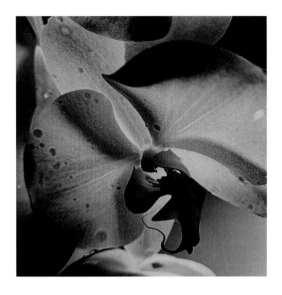

in a singleness that is faithful in celibacy. Through encountering this chaste love, Jane eventually becomes willing to bear children.

The form of this world is passing away, Paul writes, enjoining those who "have wives to live as though they had none, and those who mourn [to live] as though they were not mourning, and those who rejoice as though they were not rejoicing." (1 Cor. 7:29–31). Paul's exhortation incorporates Hannah's inversion of the sorrow of barrenness. The declaration of the gospel in the realm of procreation not only offers hope to the childless, but places a great qualifier over the joy of the fruitful: baptism is our entry into the kingdom of God, not the blessing of fertility.

A world that rejects God will reject creation. Yet the paradox is that we must look beyond creation itself if we wish to renew its authority and goodness within our communities. Life in the kingdom of God both confirms and disturbs our love of creation. To paraphrase Lewis, those who

focus on the family rather than the kingdom will eventually have neither – but those who look to the kingdom shall have family given to them as well. We announce the gospel in the realm of sex and procreation only when our exhortations to marry

> To paraphrase C. S. Lewis, those who focus on the family rather than the kingdom will eventually have neither – but those who look to the kingdom shall have family given to them as well.

and procreate honor the fact that the children who bear our name are "not the good things of the eternal Jerusalem," but are the "good things that belong to the land of the dying" – as Augustine once wrote.

The abundance of St. Anne's on the Hill is born out of the Christian tragedy of childlessness, which confirms the goods of creation by looking toward what they point to – a life of participating in the works of charity toward all those whom God gives to us to love. The endlessness of love never fails, though our hopes and dreams for our lives in this world sometimes might. God's good gifts sometimes come in strange and severe forms, yet each of them is ordered toward the perfection of our joy in the gift of our lives to God and each other. Within the economy of God's love, the barren will someday wear their crowns of triumph at the city gates. They, too, will no longer be ashamed. ⤙

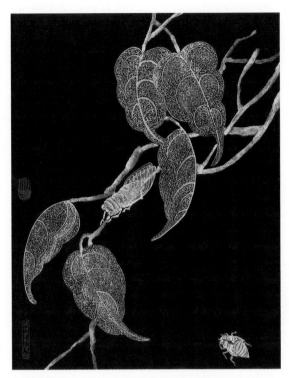

HyunJung Kim, *Prayer of a Cicada*, gold powder on paper, 2017

The Revenant

That winter when awareness flies away
and I keep losing keys and cat and mind,
time will be falling, time will fall behind
over and over, dimmer day by day.

Surprise, then, will decide the way of things,
and I won't bother over what life means.
Youth will revive at times, and playground scenes—
me in the sandbox, friends on slides and swings.

May I at least once find you on the lawn,
lie there, your spry lap holding up my head,
and worship you, since you are ten years dead
and I want to forget that you are gone.

AARON POOCHIGIAN

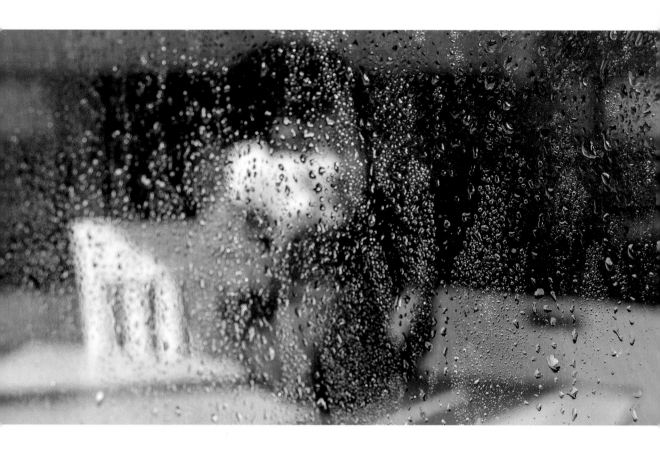

The Stranger in My House

We adopted children with trauma in their past.
It didn't go as expected.

WENDY KIYOMI

THE BEDROOM DOOR was pockmarked with fresh dents. I swung it closed, leaving it ajar, and walked the ten steps down the hall to my own room. I had just coaxed my child, who had spent four hours slamming furniture, throwing blocks at my head, and screaming expletives, finally to bed. My mind reeled from all I had heard: "Fucking asshole! I hope you stab yourself until you die, you idiot!" I sat down shakily and realized my hands were trembling. I had never felt visceral fear like this before, fear because of my own child, a child I had invited into my home and into permanent, intimate relationship by adoption.

Even though I wasn't exactly surprised by the evening's events, I felt disoriented. I had never questioned that adoption was *family,* but that evening I found myself asking, "Who is this person in my house?" Parenting under these circumstances seemed a far cry from my notion of family. It resembled something closer to hospitality.

Before our children arrived from foster care, my biggest question about inviting others into our home had to do with how much cleaning to do before guests arrived. I was cavalier about some messiness, but my husband preferred a tidy house – it was more welcoming, he said. It turned out we had glossed over the most important question of all: "Who is our guest?" Like others we knew, we were comfortable with the expected hospitality of having friends and family over. But that evening, as I shook with fear, it struck me that churchgoers rarely talk about hospitality to people who are rude or unruly. We seldom invite people who are disabled or injured, and we definitely do not have guests who are not safe.

The uncomfortable truth was that we had some unsafe people in the house, people we had invited in. In becoming their family, we had promised to love them unconditionally, and we did. But we had no practice in this kind of hospitality.

Biblically, guests are venerated and sometimes divine. "Come, Lord Jesus, be our guest" is the opening of a prayer that recognizes this. Theologian Henri J. M. Nouwen names children as our most important guests. "They enter into our homes, ask for careful attention, stay for a while, and then leave to follow their own way," he writes. Whether by birth or adoption, any child enters a family as a guest. We cannot predict beforehand exactly what hardships we sign up for when we welcome a child, but we are certain to encounter some.

We may feel that we know birthchildren before we meet them, while children who enter a family

by adoption seem defined by their strangeness. The truth is that strangeness accompanies all new arrivals. My friend anticipating a new baby put this idea to poetry: "You, the long-expected stranger, who are you to pierce my heart so wide?" To welcome any child is to enter the rich stream of hospitality that God initiated when he formed Adam and Eve, when he called Abraham in the wilderness, and when he granted David kingship. King David was a "man after God's own heart," who experienced such deep intimacy with God that he belonged to him as a child – God called him his firstborn (Ps. 89). Yet David himself was acutely aware of his guest status with the Lord, praying, "we are foreigners and strangers in your sight" (1 Chron. 29:15). Hospitality and family are closely related in the Lord's taxonomy of welcome.

AS I FACED THE PROBLEM of my child's difficult behaviors, I found that my larger problem was the flimsy theological framework that "family" alone lent to my efforts to understand and love my child. The framework of family was the preeminent concept undergirding every adoption handbook, memoir, and theological treatise in our library. It makes sense. Unattached children need a family, adoption provides one, ergo adoption is a family matter. Everyone, adoptive families included, expects adoptive families to look, feel, and act like families – without a solid understanding of what "family" might mean.

There is also an expectation that "building a family" through adoption provides a permanent solution to a child's problem. A child is family-less, then is adopted. Problem solved. This is upheld in popular narratives about adoption, such as *Anne of Green Gables.* Affectionate, eager, and motivated, Anne articulates a conscious desire for a family and has the relational skills to thrive there; truly her problem is solved when she's

---

Wendy Kiyomi is the pen name of an adoptive parent, scientist, and writer in Washington State.

matched with a family. Once she works through a few minor episodes of name-calling and slate-breaking, she is good to go as a connected and well-adjusted teenager.

In reality, children needing adoption come to their new families with profound experiences of loss. They have lost the primary relationships that are the foundation of their whole existence. Many

---

If, as psychologist Curt Thompson writes, "we are all born into the world looking for someone looking for us," many children have never found what they're looking for.

---

have additionally suffered the loss of healthy development in utero and of loving nurture in early childhood. If, as psychiatrist Curt Thompson writes, "we are all born into the world looking for someone looking for us," many children have never found what they're looking for. The early losses of "children from hard places," as developmental psychologist Karyn Purvis calls them, become a permanent physiological blueprint that gives rise to ongoing impairments in loving others, regulating their emotions, and organizing their inner selves. Such children are frequently unable to show reciprocal affection to their caregivers, which Deborah D. Gray, in her book *Attaching in Adoption*, describes as not "gratifying." A gratifying child, like Anne, instinctively shows consideration, tenderness, and a sense of exclusive attachment. Even a healthy parenting relationship is likely to entail more giving than receiving – but for caregiving to have no apparent impact on the child is quite discouraging.

I treasured the times when I could easily tell that my children needed me and regarded me with affection. My two-year-old would stop screaming and nestle in my lap when I picked her up and rubbed her back. My son would lean into me comfortably as I read *Faster, Faster! Nice and Slow!* before bedtime. He'd place his hand on my shoulder as we cooked pancakes together the next morning as mother and son. As my children grew, I delighted in their insight that showed they both knew and loved me. My daughter came downstairs the other day wearing jeans I had recently told her were a bit tight. As she walked into the kitchen and saw me gathering my energies for a lecture, she looked smilingly in my eyes, caressed my arm, and said, "Mom, you're going to be fine."

Even with such moments of tenderness, adoptive parents and children must often live as a family while not *feeling* how a family is expected to feel. Our household resembled a family in that we had the ordinary assortment of adults and children doing family activities, but we didn't feel like a family in some key ways. At a Christian conference on foster and adoptive parenting, my husband and I sat together listening to a pediatrician give a workshop titled, "Can We Get to Happy and Calm?" After we had spent ten years providing our kids with specialized parenting, intense educational accommodations, predictable routines, weekly counseling, grandparent involvement, thoughtful extracurriculars, and both parents working part time so we could be home as much as possible, the answer was apparently "no." We had been trying to be the best family we could, and it didn't work. We knew the truth of psychologist Gregory Keck's observation that children from hard places "bring their pain into their new families and share it with much vigor and regularity."

A nurturing adoptive family sometimes isn't enough to bring healing to children shaped by trauma. Children who don't heal "end up filling our jails, our welfare rolls, and our medical

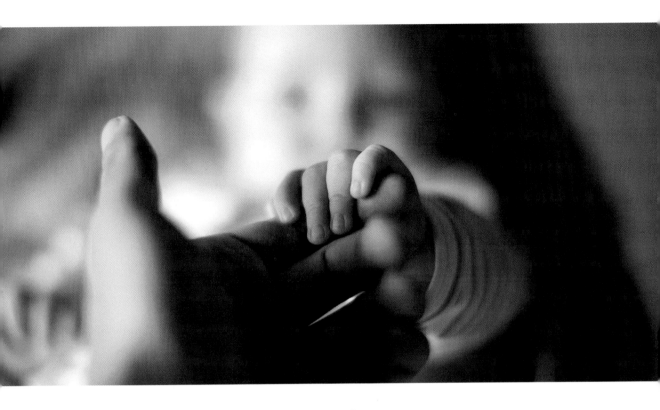

clinics," according to trauma researcher Bessel van der Kolk. Kids from hard places are wounded and vulnerable, in need of distinctively Christian hospitality that Christine Pohl describes as pressing "out toward the weakest, those least likely to be able to reciprocate."

A big part of feeling like a family today is matching the idealization of home as a wholesome retreat and of family as a healthy and mutually supportive group of loyal, like-minded individuals. Rodney Clapp, author of *Families at the Crossroads*, characterizes our culture's pervasive concept of family as private, inward-focused, and dedicated to sentiment. We are biased toward health, and we assign success only to families that match what I call Christmas card criteria, where everyone is "healthy and doing well." Unsuccessful families often take on the shame and isolation that come with failing to match these ideals.

This family framework is inherently difficult for adoptive families because the kids may be impaired and needy. But we are far from alone. Poverty, disability, chronic illness, misfortune, generational trauma, and our sinful nature complicate the realization of this ideal for so many people. An affectionate, supportive, and healthy nuclear family is a beautiful gift from God. But admiring a gift, especially when it's bestowed on someone else, can distract us from the Giver.

Moreover, when we conceptualize family only as a safe home base rich in good feelings and comfort, we stunt the family's purpose and calling. Our aim easily becomes too narrow, too fleeting, and most of all, too protectionist. Jesus predicted that in this world we would have trouble (John 16:33), and he called his followers not away from pain but toward it, provided we take courage from the right source – his victory over the world. A comfortable family ideal makes it easy to look askance at the risks of involvement with a needy and dangerous world and to justify insularity for the sake of preserving the family.

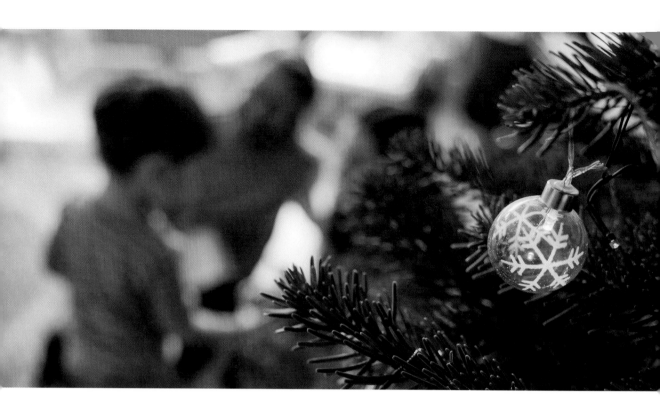

WHEN I WAS ABLE to reframe our calling as one of hospitality, it was a divine paradigm shift.

Of course, not all adopted children struggle with attachment or dangerous behavior. Many thrive in healthy homes with no such problems on the surface. But all have endured profound loss. Adoptive parents must understand that their role has to be broad enough to encompass the full range of trauma.

To practice adoption well, to do what Deborah Gray calls "the most valuable work accomplished in society" of helping children forge attachments after loss, we need a sturdier framework to enable adoptive parents to love a child despite the pain and suffering it often brings.

Considering adoption through the lens of hospitality anticipates a real encounter with suffering and offers a means of accounting for it. The primary movement of adoption is not away from brokenness but toward it; adoptive parents give it room at the very heart of their homes. Practitioners of biblical hospitality expect to suffer because they continually lay their lives down "in little pieces and small acts of sacrificial love and service," writes Pohl. This costly calling is compassion, literally "co-suffering," in which parents begin to bear not only their children's old pain but also the pain that results from a new configuration of vulnerable, fallen individuals.

Suffering can dehumanize us with its anarchy and break our hope of God's goodness. Hospitality renders suffering not less painful but instead centered in the heart of God. "God is near to lowliness," writes Dietrich Bonhoeffer; "he loves the lost, the neglected, the unseemly, the excluded, the weak and broken." When we practice hospitality toward the neediest and the weakest, by proximity we also experience the great love of God: outwardly we may be wasting away but inwardly we are being renewed day by day (2 Cor. 4:16). Christ, the ultimate host, suffered greatly. He left his honored place as adored Son, and took pain, humiliation, and death to himself on behalf of those he invites as guests. Jesus pulls the suffering of hospitality into the service of God's intentional and relentless overthrow of brokenness.

In God's economy, hospitality is never a one-sided practice in which the host does all the giving, and the guests do all the receiving. In biblical stories of hospitality, guests have a special way of connecting their hosts with God and his extravagant gifts. The Shunammite woman who kept a guest room for Elisha was thrice blessed by God in the birth of her son, his later resuscitation, and the restoration of her property. Abraham and Sarah's mysterious visitors were heralds of God's gift of a long-awaited child. Mary was the first host to the Christ Child; she cherished her unexpected pregnancy, singing that the baby's arrival was also the advent of the Lord's full mercy, justice, and abundance for herself and all people. Other hosts to Jesus, like Zacchaeus, who invited him to his house to dine, and Mary, a follower who anointed his feet with perfume, were honored beyond their deserts and given a special place in Jesus' heart and the history of the world.

Adoption as an expression of hospitality looks for the possibility of entertaining angels. This is both comforting and alarming. Biblical visits by angels are rarely serene affairs. Angels often bring difficult news, messages of what God is doing to accomplish his will, and challenging directives. But angels are a visitation by God himself.

Our adopted children have brought many blessings – the sentimental blessings of cuddling their small bodies and receiving their affection; the practical blessings of bringing me into contact with our community and other families for support and friendship; even the psychological blessings of developing my emotional intelligence and discovering my own neediness. But the main

blessing is that to parent them is to rush headlong into the presence and love of Christ.

The very experiences that are the most painful are the ones that give me the most personal encounter with Christ's love for the world in general and my family in particular. This is often not the blessing I want – sacrificial love sounds beautiful, but it is not nice. Sacrificial love is an

---

Adoption as an expression of hospitality looks for the possibility of entertaining angels. This is both comforting and alarming.

---

emptying process; it strips us of things we hold dear, even our agency, our very ability to influence events or control our environment. Somehow, though, this love is the means to experiencing the devastating beauty of the love of Christ.

Jesus was a princely host who also relied on others to continually supply his needs. His risky hospitality did not occur apart from regular displays of neediness as a vulnerable stranger and guest. Biblical hospitality joins the expressions of hosting and guesting, bringing us into childlike dependence on our Father. Christine Pohl explains that "this intermingling of guest and host roles in the person of Jesus is part of what makes the story of hospitality so compelling for Christians." Framing adoption as an intersection of guest and host strengthens all parents, adoptive or not, by barring the treacherous path of self-sufficiency. To the extent that Jesus our Savior and ultimate host was dependent on the provision of others, so parents can openly practice Christlike dependence on their God, friends, and even strangers.

I REACHED A POINT in parenting where I did not, because I could not, conceal my feelings of poverty. Somehow all my yearnings were at the surface. I missed a call one day from the Christian high school principal and had to call him back. I dreaded a sermon, perhaps with allusions to the Church Fathers, about my child's behavior. I was surprised when I started telling him about my child's losses and impairments, and even more surprised when he responded with empathy and hope. He did quote Augustine: "Since love grows within you, so beauty grows," bringing tears to my eyes. The friendships and divine appointments that have arisen from sharing my fragility with others have been my best joys and firmest assurance of God's personal concern for me.

Risky hospitality is different from recklessness. Violence or danger in the home is serious, and biblical hospitality to one guest must not endanger other members of the household. A hospitality framework charters its own limits. We may be tempted to think that a family will do anything for its children, and when the goals are to secure comfort and affection, parents can easily assume responsibility for the family's entire psychological environment in addition to how the kids "turn out." My friend Annie has five children, and she articulated to me the mental exhaustion and emotional heaviness of this kind of striving. "I can do a good job loving and caring for my kids," she said, "but I can't analyze and correct all the interactions everywhere in the household."

Jesus healed some but not all; his calling was not a rush to reach every sick person immediately. In Christlike hospitality, we recognize that much brokenness will go unremedied for now, and our call is to generously offer what we can while fostering a trust in God's nature as redeemer and healer. This is how we may sacrificially love without losing our souls. It isn't ours to fix our guest but to keep a place where we watch for what God will do. The tenets of hospitality can help us see what care we can wisely provide in our home and when, like the Good Samaritan, we need to turn the care over to others.

Hospitality has grounded my emotions, actions, thoughts, and prayers regarding our children – all that constitutes discipleship – in the alternating guestness and hostness of Christ. Within that framework is his mysterious love that shapes me to be the parent I need to be for my needy little strangers. The fruit of hospitality is sometimes painfully unseen and sometimes astonishingly beautiful.

My teenage children all still let me put them to bed. Recently I went to tuck in my son whose distress and challenges leading up to bedtime were so difficult for everyone. He needed much more than a cozy goodnight, but that was all I had to offer. I asked him how he wanted me to pray for him.

"I dunno," he said, "maybe for a good day tomorrow."

As I prayed, I felt his shoulders twitch a couple of times – he was falling asleep. At the end, his eyes fluttered open, and he asked, "Can you sing that other song real quick?"

"Which other song?" I asked. "All Praise to Thee My God This Night?"

"Yeah," he said.

My heart was heavy, but I sang to him:

All praise to thee, my God, this night,
For all the blessings of the light;
Keep me, O keep me, King of kings,
Beneath thine own almighty wings.

He was asleep by the second stanza. Those verses were a prayer, that the King of kings would keep both of us in his protection and in the light that shines in the darkness. Whether I was host or guest in that sacred moment, I do not know; God knows.

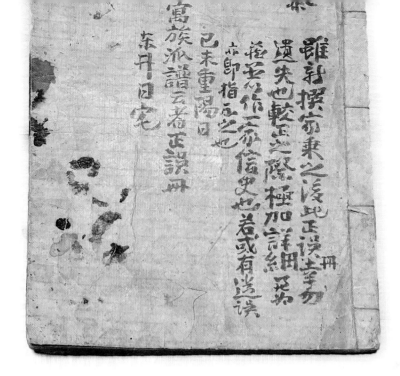

The Name of My
Forty-Sixth-Great-Grandfather

My children are growing up far from our ancestral village in Korea. An ancient book connects them back.

JAEHYOUNG JEONG

H E HASN'T ADDED my children's names yet. But in a few years, my father will take his family registry, all of two inches thick, to get updated and reprinted. When he does, it will trace my family's story in an unbroken line from my youngest child and only daughter, Jimene Jeong 정지민, an American citizen, back forty-nine generations to DukSung Jeong 정덕성, the first Korean citizen in our family.

Many Korean families have registry books like this. Confucianism is the dominant religious philosophy of the country; respect and honor toward our ancestors is central to our culture. Not all families keep up their books and databases

Jaehyoung 정재형 and Hyeyoung 전혜영 Jeong moved to the Bruderhof in 2015 from South Korea. They have four sons and a daughter and live at the Fox Hill community in New York State.

The Jeongs' hand-lettered book of genealogical records.

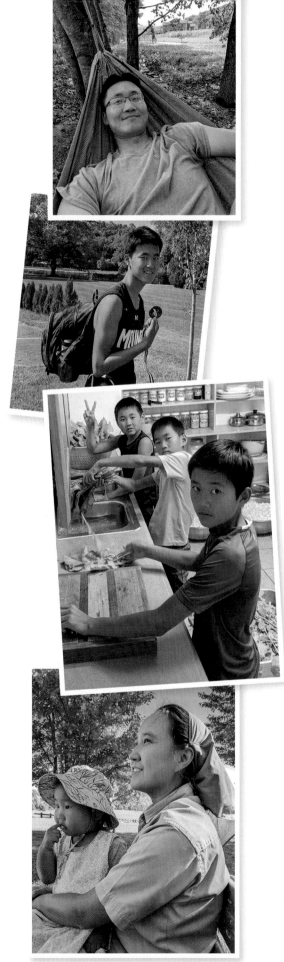

religiously. But for most it's a sacred duty. Within our Jeong family, there are five main "limbs" of our tree that over the centuries have branched out in hundreds of directions. Our clan now has more than 200,000 people. Of course we are scattered far and wide, and do not all remain in touch. One of the main family "limbs" considers it their right or duty to maintain a website with much of the collective history, as well as marriages, births, and deaths – as many as they are informed of.

And in print form, we have that beautiful book, with names and birthdates flowing vertically down and to the left, across page after page. On the shelf next to the print version, there's the more fragile brush and ink, hand-lettered volume, to speak for earlier centuries. Growing up, I never gave these books more than a passing glance. I played and studied in the shadow of my ancestors' names and stories without giving them more thought and care than was their familial due.

So why, now that I can only view their distant pages digitally, from half a world away, do I take such note of my father's name, of mine and my brother's, and the space that will soon mark the existence of my children? Why do I find myself looking much farther back, as far back in the pages as it's possible to look, and reading the story of another transplant, who took his family into a new and unexpected life?

N AD 853, DukSung Jeong, a trusted official in the Chinese government with a high position in the Ministry of National Defense, had a falling out with the emperor and was exiled to the small island of Aphaedo 압해도 on the southwest coast of Korea.

The family history tells us that he and his family found a welcome there, so much so that he chose to stay and adopt a new homeland, even when the winds at court changed and he was invited back to resume his governmental duties in China.

His grave and memorial house still stand on the island where he made his new home and started

Top to bottom: Jaehyoung Jeong; his oldest son, Yeoho; Yechan, Darvell, and Ihreh; and his wife, Hyeyoung, with their daughter, Jimene.

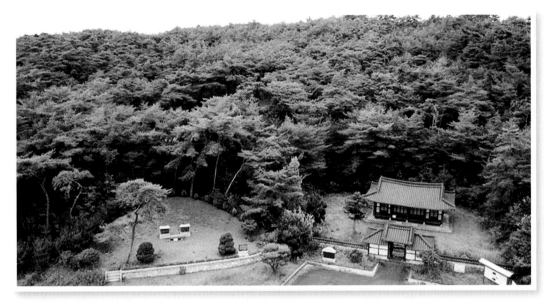

The memorial site of DukSung Jeong in South Korea

our Korean family. Across almost 1,200 years, I feel more related to him than I do to my nearer ancestors. I know that we share a birthday, after all – October 13. I should like to ask him how he navigated such a big cultural shift with his family. Did he struggle with a new language, as I still do? What did he miss about home? What most made him want to stay? What did he teach his children about their roots? What would he want me to teach mine?

Perhaps my family will stand there one day, on the land that became his home and therefore ours. I will stand there for a long time. Then I will take my wife and children to meet relatives who live near this island, so we can hear more stories of the people who came before us, because not everything is written down.

I OWE MY ANCESTORS a depth of respect that I struggle to put into words for my children, whether in our native language that my wife and I strive to keep them fluent in, or in English where we struggle to keep up with them.

I am a Christian, so I do not worship my forebears as is customary in Confucian households. But I would like my five children to understand that if they do not know where they come from,

they cannot know where they are going. Multiple generations each contributed something precious and valuable to those of us alive now. The links build on each other. They should not be broken now because people have forgotten.

We are not just dropped from the air. In Genesis, we read Ruth's family tree. It goes back to Adam, then to God. My family tree book, along with everyone else's, written and unwritten, has parallels to Genesis. This is my root, my source, which goes back – eventually – to God. God is present in the stories of all the ancestors.

That is what I want to pass on to my children. They were born Korean, and we are a Korean family, but now they live in an American community – a different culture, a different language. There will be confusing times ahead for them; perhaps not right now, but when they are teenagers, when they grow up and start families of their own. But if they know who they are, the depth of their roots, the story of their history, it can hold them. I would like to tell them: even though you are different from others, even though your parents are quite different from the parents of others, it's okay. Your roots run deep, and you are the next generation, the next page in an ancient book. ⌁

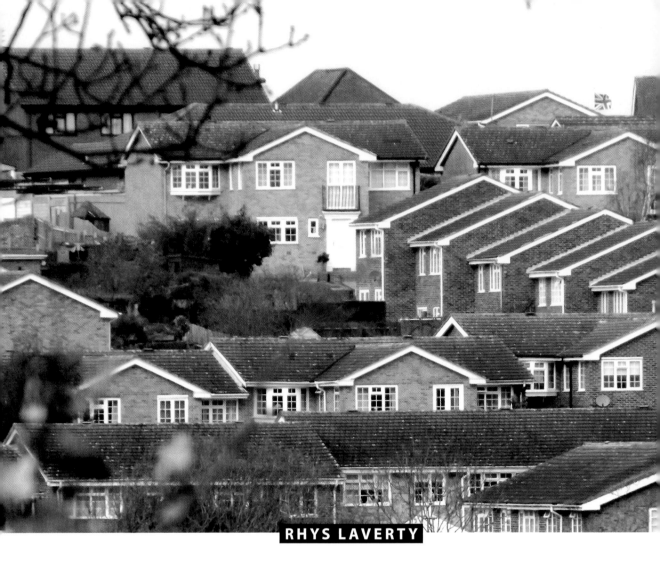

RHYS LAVERTY

Somewhere in Chessington

My hometown debunks the idea that family-friendly neighborhoods are a thing of the past.

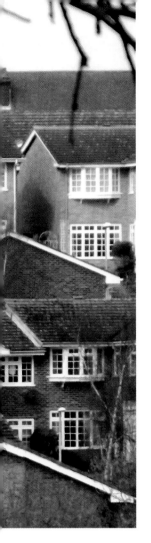

Early last summer, Mum called to say she'd be having a minor operation that would take her out of action for six weeks. Swiftly, that ugly modern crisis was upon me: *childcare*. Mum looks after our kids twice a week – what would we do?

"Don't worry," said Mum, "it's sorted."

And it was. When I started explaining things to my wife, she blurted out "What about childcare?" I leaned over and repeated a mantra of ours: "*Trust the herd.*" For six weeks, the kids bounced between two of their great-aunts, with my cousins on standby, and even my dad valiantly chipping in. I hadn't even needed to make a telephone call.

When I've told the story since, the response is always the same: "You're so lucky – so few people have that nowadays." And that seems true. Of my close university friends, only I returned home to live in the same town as my family. For those friends, intergenerational relationships happen maybe at Christmas. For me, it's day-to-day. Yet in the grand sweep of history and geography, I'm not particularly unusual. In most places, and at most times, successive generations stay put. It's not that *nobody* moved around before the twentieth century – wind the clock back to, say, the fourteenth century, and you'd find a lot of Flemish artisans and tradesmen knocking around England looking for work. But, by and large, human beings have tended to stay put with their elders and offspring.

But that's changed in the United Kingdom. An Ancestry survey in 2017 showed that Britons now live on average 100 miles away from where they were born. A generation ago, the average was five miles. Just one-third of people live in their childhood home, and only half still live nearby. Newspaper reports at the time strangely claimed that this showed the desire to move away was "not overwhelming," which seems a bit "glass half full" to me. My hometown, Chessington, seems to be (just about) bucking this trend – something for which I'm very grateful. But I'm worried about how long it will stay that way.

By rights, Chessington should have long since dissolved indistinctly into the suburban sprawl of London's Zone 6. But quirks of roadbuilding give it some surprisingly definite borders: the M25 hems the south; the A3 divides us north and west from leafy Surbiton (made famous by *The Good Life*); eastward, everyone knows that once you're past the Jet garage on Ruxley Lane, you're into Epsom and Ewell. And so it remains, despite its affluent neighbors, a working-class redoubt of just under twenty thousand souls, largely the families of what an outsider might call "white-van men" – builders, plumbers, and electricians. Whether or not they drive vans, they tend to work with their hands, love their wives and kids, and enjoy a drink after work down the pub (of which we have many – nearly double the national average ratio of pubs to people, in fact).

Chessington is moderately famous for its zoo and World of Adventures theme park. Others say its best feature is having two train stations – twice as many chances to leave! But, for whatever reason, people tend to stay put. It's the kind of place where you know your friends' parents and your parents' friends. I am not the only person here with more aunts than Bertie Wooster.

Rhys Laverty is senior editor of Ad Fontes Journal *and managing editor at the Davenant Press. He lives in Chessington, United Kingdom, with his wife, Libby, daughter, Noah, and son, Seamus.*

Chessington from the South, 2012. Photograph by Colin Smith.

In 2017, David Goodhart published *The Road to Somewhere: The Populist Revolt and the Future of Politics*. Goodhart was pegged as one of the "Brexit whisperers," a translator of the disaffected working classes. He framed national divisions as primarily between the "Anywheres" and the "Somewheres." The Anywheres derive their identities from intangibles such as their education and careers; the Somewheres derive theirs from a sense of place and local community.

The Anywheres are not new, exactly. Aristotle remarked on the theoretical dangerousness of someone without a state. In his *Politics*, he says that "he who by nature and not by mere accident is without a state, is either a bad man or above humanity; he is like the 'tribeless, lawless, heartless one' whom Homer denounces – the natural outcast is forthwith a lover of war; he may be compared to an isolated piece at draughts." The Anywheres seem particularly ascendant these days, so Goodhart's categories are useful not just for thinking about Brexit, but for understanding twenty-first-century Britain more broadly. The key reason, I think, that Chessington remains a highly intergenerational town is that it is still populated by working-class Somewheres: if you stick around in a place, you can't help but form bonds between old and young, within your family and without.

How did Chessington get this way? You can trace the place back to Anglo-Saxon days, but for a long time it was just a hamlet, outside the slightly more substantial village of Hook (to this day, one of my mum's more aspirational friends insists she lives in Hook, *not* Chessington). Chessington really began to develop as a town after the zoo's founding in 1931, soon subsuming Hook. Rows of newbuilds went up, along with the train line to London built in 1939. The post–World War II suburban boom took it from strength to strength: half an hour from Waterloo by rail, with good road connections into London, it provided ample work opportunities, growing into a thriving working-class town, insulated from London and Surrey on either side.

By the mid-1960s, it was an ideal place to settle down, which is exactly what all my grandparents did. Dave and Pat, my maternal grandparents, were local already (the house Dave was born in is five minutes from mine); the welfare state was in its prime, and both worked in the National Health Service, allowing them to buy their family home in 1966. My paternal grandparents, Dan and Maud, hailed from Ireland and the Channel Islands. After serving in the Royal Navy, Grandad Dan could never return to Ireland for fear of Republican reprisals. He and my grandmother met during the war and, after grandad's career brought him to Surrey in the late sixties, Chessington became their home. UK homebuilding peaked around this time, and he and my granny bought a house on one of several new estates. Granny remained proud for years that theirs had been the show home for the whole estate – so proud, it seems, she didn't change a thing. After they died fifty years later, we discovered they'd not once updated the wiring.

In my parents' lifetimes, various other circumstances helped keep Chessington a stable place for family life. In 1980, Margaret Thatcher introduced the "Right to Buy," allowing people to buy their council homes (of which there were an abundance – council housing encompassed more than 30 percent of homes in the seventies). Despite being opposed to the policy in principle, my dad (like almost everyone else) couldn't turn down the offer. Transportation improved as well: in 1985 Chessington joined the M25 with the completion of Junction 9, opening up a new world of work for my dad as a haulage and demolition driver who eventually set up his own business. Proximity to London always meant prices were somewhat higher than elsewhere – two of my aunts had to move out to get on the property ladder before getting back in. But having been populated by working-class folk in the preceding decades, and then filled with large amounts of council housing, the town resisted anything resembling gentrification.

So, bit by bit, Chessington became a highly intergenerational place. Dave, Pat, Dan, and Maud all died here, each pair leaving behind four children. Today, three of each set still live here, as do most of their children (and their growing number of grandchildren). They are my aunts, uncles, cousins, nephews, and nieces. I can barely leave the house without bumping into one of them. Almost all these people could be fairly described

afford to raise their families here. In many places, when house prices rise, owners sell up and move on, usually to a more prosperous neighborhood. Not here. Chessington is surrounded by leafier, more affluent areas – Surbiton, Claygate, Epsom – but no Chessingtonian in his right mind wants to live in such poncy places. Working-class people don't want to move to middle-class places; they want to stay where they are but with more

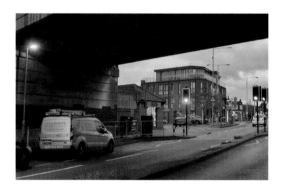

Chessington remains a working-class redoubt of just under twenty thousand souls, largely the families of what an outsider might call "white-van men" – builders, plumbers, electricians.

as Somewheres. Perhaps my family is a bit bigger than some others, but most folk in Chessington are a lot like us. This is their Somewhere; their values in life are shaped primarily by what goes on *here*, not in Westminster or New York or Los Angeles. Their families, like mine, have been around for a while, so their intergenerational networks involve not only family members but the countless mates-of and ex-boyfriend's-mums-of that they can't help but acquire. This is why you will often find eighteen-year-olds drinking in the pub with their mum's friends.

So what's changing? My fear is that this town of Somewheres may be, unwittingly, turning itself into one of Anywheres.

Two things, above all else, threaten the demise of intergenerational families here: house prices and higher education.

House prices are a national problem, nowhere more than in London and its fringe. Like everywhere else, Boomers and Gen-Xers bought property when times were good, so they could

money. Rather than a new house, money goes to improving the one you already have. My church's new pastor remarked in a sermon recently that he'd never seen a town with so many loft conversions – and it's true.

Yet the children of these Boomer and Gen-X homeowners now struggle to afford to live here. Two of my cousins, both with children of their own, have had to move in with their parents to save for a house. Others I know have had to uproot themselves to somewhere cheaper to start their own families, turning intergenerational relationships once maintained on a daily basis into the stuff of WhatsApp groups and bank-holiday visits. When their parents eventually die, having likely sold their house to pay for their final years in a nursing home, inflated house prices (exacerbated by the expensive elaboration of loft conversions and extensions) mean there's no way their children will be able to afford what were once their parents' homes. A bubble seems set to burst: when the affluent working-class Boomers start dying or selling their homes to pay for care, an affluent middle-class commuter set will arrive in force, likely gentrifying the place, driving prices up even more, and killing off a working-class town once and for all. The younger generations will be scattered to who knows where, like the exiled Cockneys of Essex.

Then there's education. In *The Road to Somewhere*, Goodhart observes that the "helter-skelter expansion of higher education" and "the elevation of educational success as the main

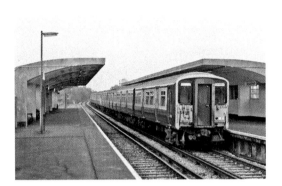

marker of social esteem" since the early 1990s have powered the triumph of Anywhere values over Somewhere values in British society. The Further and Higher Education Act 1992 doubled the number of universities in Britain by turning all polytechnic colleges into universities. Before then, the polys were largely associated with STEM qualifications, but after chafing at the snobbery of the established universities, they gradually developed their own creative and humanities degrees. The merits of the 1992 Act are still debated, but it undoubtedly led to an explosive increase in university attendance that continues to this day. Between 1992 and 2016, UK university attendance nearly doubled. Its impact is measurable by me: 1992 is the year I was born, and I was the first person on my mother's side of the family to go to university.

The prospectus of our local girls' comprehensive school boasts of its sixth form that "the vast majority of students receive the maximum five

'offers' from their chosen universities and most are accepted on to their 'first choice' of university course." One thing this means is that many of these girls won't return home. They'll stay in their uni town, move abroad, or move a few travel zones north into London proper. Those who do return will have immensely weakened their bonds with the place; they're likely to view homecoming as a kind of defeat. And you can understand why. Before they go to university, the stories of a thousand-and-one films and songs drip-feed into

Christians, who know all too well from the Garden of Eden what happens when man reaches beyond his limits, should really be the biggest Somewheres of all.

teenagers' minds something I call "Born To Run Syndrome": *"Oh, baby this town rips the bones from your back / It's a death trap, it's a suicide rap / We gotta get out while we're young / 'Cause tramps like us, baby we were born to run."* Chessington is hardly the kind of derelict East-Jesus-Nowhere that inspired Springsteen in the seventies, but the well-trodden "let's blow this popcorn stand!" myth is so ingrained by now that it may as well be. The political and ideological chemistry of university, too, is pure acid to familial bonds, invested as it is in questioning anything inherited, culture not least. Most young people don't stand a chance of developing a healthy relationship to hearth and hometown. Anywhereism makes great inroads this way.

Yet the real tragedy is that this corrosion of intergenerational working-class bonds seems, for the large part, self-inflicted. The Somewheres unknowingly, yet willingly, are handing their

Chessington North Station, 1985. Photograph by Ben Brooksbank.

children over to the Anywheres. Despite the explosion of university attendance in the last thirty years, it's still often a badge of honor for many working-class families to send a child to university, so they enthusiastically encourage their children into it. Such working-class aspiration can be a poisoned chalice, as Somewhere parents drive their children into the arms of the Anywheres. It is dispiriting to see the many teenagers I know ferried unquestioningly along the conveyor belt to university, forever weakening their bonds at home – all for the sake of (in most cases) a dubiously useful degree.

Often, their grandparents found their Somewhere here; their parents grew up here close to siblings and cousins; they probably did too. But that's changed. Despite contentment with their own lot, working-class parents often nurse an aspirational streak that supposes that somehow it's "better" for their children to go off to university. This aspirational streak is exploited by secondary schools, who marshal all their resources to funnel children toward university, since more kids at university looks better for the school. Just before Christmas, my wife, a teacher at a local boys' state secondary school, had a sixth-former go missing overnight. He turned up the next day, distressed and scruffy after a night's wandering. He'd had a minor breakdown because of the pressure to apply to university – which he didn't want to do. This is the other way Anywhereism wins: through the Somewheres' suicide by aspiration.

What becomes of these Somewhere-cum-Anywheres, wherever they end up? Some outcomes are obvious. If they have kids, grandparents are often a long way away, and there is just no replacement for having grandparents close by. But it's about more than that: what of aunts, cousins, uncles, neighbors – those less well-defined, gloriously unscripted familial and extrafamilial relationships whose great strength is their lack of definition, leaving more room for the abundance of personality than those of parents or grandparents?

Dylan Thomas wrote, "There are always uncles at Christmas" – gorgeously true, but why not all year round? Who can estimate the value of bumping into an uncle (unrelated to you by blood) at the shops, and him, unprompted, giving you a beefy kiss on the cheek, telling you "Don't worry about the kids, mister, you're a great dad"?

My mum attended the aforementioned girls' comprehensive in the seventies, and she recalls that "hardly anybody went to university." She didn't. Nor did any of her friends. She lives literally over the road from her old school and has never really gone anywhere else. She turned sixty this year and is holding two separate parties – the first for ladies only. She invited one hundred people, ranging from teenagers to women in their eighties. My cousins' friends were there – because my mum has known them all their lives. Will any of those girls now applying successfully for their five university choices be able to throw a sixtieth birthday party like that? I doubt it.

As a Christian, I'm inevitably faced with the question of what the witness of the church should be in a town sliding from Somewhere to Anywhere. On one level, there is an instinctive Christian reaction of unconcern – after all, our home is heaven; we are but poor wayfaring strangers traveling here below; in Christ there is neither Jew nor Gentile, slave nor free, Chessingtonian nor Londoner. Considered this way, Christians may seem, on the earthly plane, the most Anywhere folk of all, our only Somewhere being the new creation. Yet grace does not destroy nature but perfects it. God has marked out our appointed times in history and the boundaries of our lands, and commands us to remain as we were when we were called. In an age that rejects the givens of human nature, there seem few greater imperatives for the church than to be a stickler for humanity. Considered this way, Christians, who know all too well from the Garden of Eden what happens when man reaches beyond his limits, should really be the biggest Somewheres of all. ⇀

Singing the Law

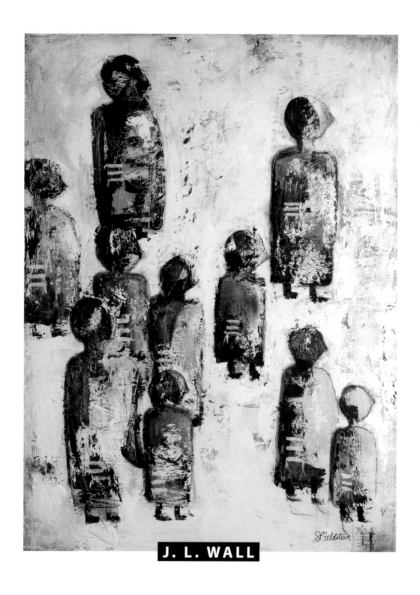

J. L. WALL

*Chanting the Torah joins past generations
to generations yet unborn.*

MY SECOND DAUGHTER arrived on her own schedule, gradually and then suddenly: eight days late, an induced labor in which nothing seemed to happen for twenty-four hours while I paced and read while my wife waited more patiently – and then, there she was.

I spent the weeks before her birth pacing the house and fidgeting in my chair. I was eager for her arrival, of course, but this need to burn impatient energy was also my reaction to an absence. I wasn't spending my free evening hours learning the Torah reading for the coming week – and I could, somehow, feel this in the muscles of my arms.

Jews have gathered to hear the Torah read aloud since the time of Ezra the Scribe, at the return from the Babylonian exile, when the people assembled to hear him read. This was a moment of refounding a nation, of reforging a link across the generations after a half-century of exile. What came after could not be the same, exactly, as that which preceded it: the Judaism that followed could not help but be more aware of its precarity.

The role of the Torah changed too. Not only a historical record or a code of laws, it also became a document to be *performed* in the hope that this might help ensure continuity from one generation to the next.

And so reading from the Torah stands at the center of Shabbat morning services in all denominations of Judaism. Learning to do this reading – or *leyning*, as it's commonly called (from the Yiddish *leyenen*, "to read") – has, in its turn, become the central element of bar and bat mitzvah study that lead to Jewish adulthood. Most of us, of course, do not go on to become a *ba'al kriyah*, a Torah reader; few ever *leyn*

again. Chalk this up to just another failure of American Judaism: we treat bar mitzvah study as preparation for checking a box, not an ethic that permeates the life to come.

I write this as one of those failures: the star Hebrew-school student at a suburban Reform synagogue who could grasp the language faster than anyone else but who had a tin ear and couldn't read the sheet music the rabbis placed in front of me. I checked the bar mitzvah box. Time passed; I drifted toward Modern Orthodoxy, where the lengthy Torah readings, on an annual rather than triennial schedule, were even more daunting.

Leyning is an acquired skill and a time-consuming task, one of the reasons that non-Orthodox denominations no longer read the full Torah portion each week. In Orthodox synagogues, it's a community effort to read the Torah in part because it *has* to be: if you want your rabbi to do any of the other tasks associated with the job, he simply can't cover all the *leyning*.

This is because, despite its name, the practice doesn't just involve reading. The text of each week's Torah portion is chanted according to a precise cantillation system (*trop* in Yiddish, *te'amim* in Hebrew). And this isn't as simple as learning a new song each week, or applying a comfortable melody to new words. The text is prose – and, as contained within a Torah scroll, without either vowels or cantillation markers. Individual *te'amim* signal not a single note, but a distinct sequence, some easy and some more complex, at times placing a dozen notes on a single syllable. At others, they require you to know variations based on the sequence in which they appear. There are patterns that grow familiar with practice, but there aren't true melodies.

J. L. Wall is the author of Situating Poetry: Covenant and Genre in American Modernism *(Johns Hopkins University Press, 2022).*

I learned to pray in Hebrew and, inconsistently, to set aside time to study the Talmud's intermingled Hebrew and Aramaic. But the Bible remained, for me, an English book.

THE COLLEGE TOWN I call home is not the wilderness of anything except Orthodox Judaism, and summers at shul are especially sparse once the students leave campus.

By the summer of 2021, our pandemic policies had burned out the members who regularly read Torah, led services, or simply showed up on time for *minyan*, the quorum of ten required to hold services. To others, the new rules gave permission for apathy. Fright thinned our numbers even further. Some families simply moved away. It was under these circumstances that I agreed to serve as the shul's interim president as we tried to pull ourselves out of Covid-induced doldrums.

One of the first tasks that fell to me in my misguided summer on a synagogue board was calling congregants late in the week to ask them to take on even more *leyning.* "This isn't easy," one of them, a talented man who has taken on more than his share for decades now, explained: "I spend hours and *hours* preparing every week." He sighed, then took on an unfairly large set of readings: shul must go on.

And that, more or less, is also how I was drawn back to *leyning* two decades after my bar mitzvah. Shul had to go on; the Torah needed to be read, so I sat teaching myself to do what had, in adolescence, felt impossible. (And still, among my community's handful of regular Torah readers, I am the least melodious and least capable.)

A year later, as our summer ranks thinned again, I couldn't guarantee that I'd be in shul, since I was awaiting the birth of my second daughter. Even if it left a significant burden on the few others available to *leyn*, I couldn't make the commitment.

So I paced. I could feel the absence in my forearms. It was physical.

IT'S A STRANGE PRACTICE, this almost-singing of the Torah. If you ask why it's done, the first answer you're likely to hear is that it clarifies the grammar. Hebrew is written without vowels; as it appears in a Torah scroll, it's also without punctuation. Naturally, this creates ambiguity, even for the fluent readers who have been a minority in Jewish history. Torah *trop* – the *te'amim* – signal which syllable should be stressed and which words link together in syntactic units; they clarify where verses begin and end.

To take one example from the *Sh'ma*: The first passage from Deuteronomy that the prayer includes begins, in English, "You will love the Lord your God." But the word as it appears in written Hebrew, even with vowels included, still might mean two very different things depending on how the word is pronounced. V'*ahav*ta is perfect: "And you loved." V'ahav*ta*, stressed on the final syllable, is imperfect: "You will love." The role of the *te'amim* is to ensure the correct and precise reading of the Torah, to maintain the continuity of its meaning from week to week and generation to generation.

That's important. But it doesn't really answer the question: Why *sing*? After all, other languages have found systems for clarifying ambiguity that don't require cantillation. Why not simply memorize the correct accentual stress, rather than a fairly elaborate set of notes?

One answer is beautification. The monks of medieval Europe did not simply copy texts but made them beautiful through calligraphy and illumination. Similarly, a talented *ba'al kriyah* illuminates the text of the Torah in the way that he reads it – my shul's rabbi emeritus is a wonderful tenor who uses his voice not for his own acclaim but to express the beauty of Torah itself. But what of a friend of mine, widely acknowledged as a skilled *ba'al kriyah*, whose voice might be generously described as atonal?

Another answer is memorization: the music aids in the accurate memorization and recitation of the words, both on a weekly basis and across generations. This should ring true: songs are easier to memorize than prose. We can find examples of this across languages and throughout history: the consistent rhythms of oral poetry, for example, may well beautify it – but they also aid in both its composition and memorization.

Jewish tradition locates the origins of this explanation within the Bible itself. The medieval exegete Rashi, for example, glosses a passage from the Talmud (*Eruvin* 21b) to credit Solomon with the creation of a system of notation for transmitting *te'amim*. *Nedarim* 21b cites Rabbi Yitzchak, who holds that the *te'amim* are the "law of Moses from Sinai": that is to say, are not just a *way* of reading Torah, but are themselves a *part* of the Oral Torah.

These answers bring us back to Judaism's awareness of its own precarity. It's not just that, in every generation, there will be those who seek to destroy us. Even without this, Judaism would have faced a crisis of transmission, the need to preserve sacred texts through an initially oral tradition.

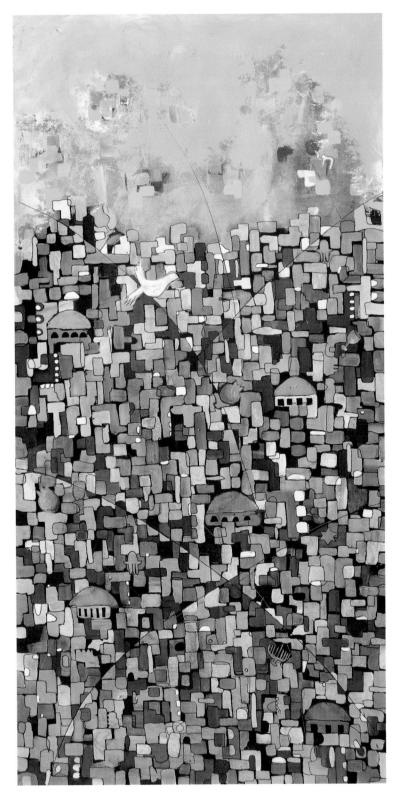

Sharon Feldstein, *O, Jerusalem no. 2*, acrylic on wood, 2022.

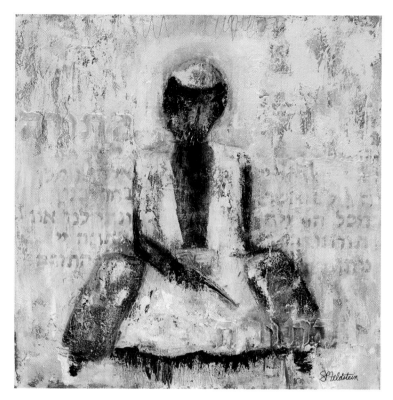

automatically," whose heads know when to bow and knees to bend, I recognize myself.

Perhaps my own shortcomings can reveal something about the purpose of the *te'amim*, as a thing worthy in itself of being passed on. Though far from ideal, Rabbi Berkovits notes, "it is no small achievement to have taught the lips to 'pray' on their own, without the conscious participation of the heart and mind . . . they too represent a form of submission of the organic self to the will to pray." "The prayer of man," he writes elsewhere in the same essay, "Law and Morality in Jewish Tradition," "should be human and not angelic," physical and embodied and not merely "in one's heart."

In other words – and this is my own extrapolation from prayer to *leyning* – perhaps we sing the Torah because it is a way to involve the fullness of our bodies in reciting and transmitting it. Perhaps, in addition to clarifying grammar, syntax, and meaning, *leyning*'s very purpose is also to force us to attend to the shape of the words in our mouths, to attune not just our minds but our diaphragms to those moments where the syntax pauses and we can breathe naturally.

My Hebrew is limited and I am shaky enough as a singer that I struggle to consciously hold both the fullness of meaning and the right *trop* in my head at once. As with my distracted prayer, this is less than ideal – but, I hope, serves a purpose. I live too much in my own head. I'm drawn to abstraction, the disinterested study that is

Most oral traditions lend themselves to the gradual transformation of their texts, but the gift of holy scripture is not meant to be so flexible.

So, why *sing* the *Law*? None of these explanations fully answers that question. Each treats the *te'amim* as a tool, a set of practices to ensure accuracy and to beautify. Chanting the Torah is part of the performance that joins generations week to week and year to year. But the *te'amim* are not just a means. As Rabbi Yitzchak insists, they are not simply a vehicle for Torah but are themselves Torah. They, too, are transmitted from week to week.

I'M NOT GOOD AT PRAYER. My mind wanders; I struggle to maintain the kind of intentionality and awareness that Judaism calls *kavana*. When the mid-century Modern Orthodox philosopher and rabbi Eliezer Berkovits writes of those whose "lips – apparently guided unconsciously – continue to form the words

Sharon Feldstein, *Reading from the Torah*, acrylic on canvas, 2020.

academic life. The risk is that my interest in Torah grows purely (even largely) intellectual: too much a part of my decidedly English-speaking mind.

When I *leyn*, I care no less about the words of the Torah; if anything, I care more. This can't be separated from the fact that when I *leyn*, I can't linger on the meaning because I'm too busy lingering on how the words themselves feel on my tongue, stretched along the notes of the *te'amim*. And it's only through this physical and embodied interaction that I'm able to encounter the Torah as Hebrew.

Still, *leyning* isn't quite song – and neither is its recitation of the written Torah the actual fulfillment of the *mitzvot* that are the true melody of Jewish life.

I like to think that in both its sound and its function, *leyning* is like recitative, those portions of opera and musical theater that are not quite sung but also not exactly spoken. The less glamorous cousin of the aria, recitative communicates the information that builds toward a fully sung climax or response. In an example Leonard Bernstein once gave, recitative passes on information like, "The price of chicken is up three cents a pound." Or – to use an example from my own *leyning* – the number of souls in subsections of the tribe of Levi.

Calling *leyning* and the weekly recitation of the written Torah "recitative" might sound diminishing. It's anything but. The analogy reveals something further – about Judaism, about observance, about the physical practice of *leyning*. In this analogy, two of the central acts of Jewish life are moments not of song but of that which precedes it, of recitative: both Sinai – the first giving of the Torah – and the Shabbat reading of the Torah, which inevitably draws the largest shul crowd of the week and for many is a key communal component of observance. Recitative builds toward a response: a choice, a decision, an action.

At Sinai, that response was, "We will do and we will hear."

But the moment of recitative repeats, week in and week out, highlighting the central drama of Jewish life: the question, again and again, in ways both mundane and significant, of whether to fulfill the *mitzvot*.

This lives in Torah reading, and in learning and teaching others to *leyn*, we transmit that drama across generations. We're taught that every Jewish soul was at Sinai – but what, exactly, does that mean? Perhaps it says something about the eternity of *that moment*, that it can continue to live in every Jewish choice and action.

Leyning transmits that moment from past to present, *l'dor v'dor*, from generation to generation. But it also prepares us for it from present to future, attuning the body as well as the mind to the words of Torah, in preparation for assent.

WHEN I HAD to step away from *leyning*, my mind missed the hours of preparation only in the abstract: I knew, as a concept, that it was a more valuable way to spend that time than scrolling Twitter or (even) poring over the expected and actual batting statistics of various Chicago Cubs infielders.

But my body *felt* the absence and longed to return.

Sitting in the hospital on the day after my daughter's birth, I realized that I had, without thinking about it, begun to scan the open *aliyot* for that week, wondering absently if I could learn one in the next two days. I couldn't – not for that Shabbat, at least. (But the week after, well, *that* was more plausible.)

We named her for the Hebrew word meaning "song," and spoke to the congregation about her name and our family. None of the words written here were among those I said; there was plenty to tell without them.

Yet I can't help but believe that all this, too, is contained in her name, is what preceded it, is what helped bring her to be. ⤴

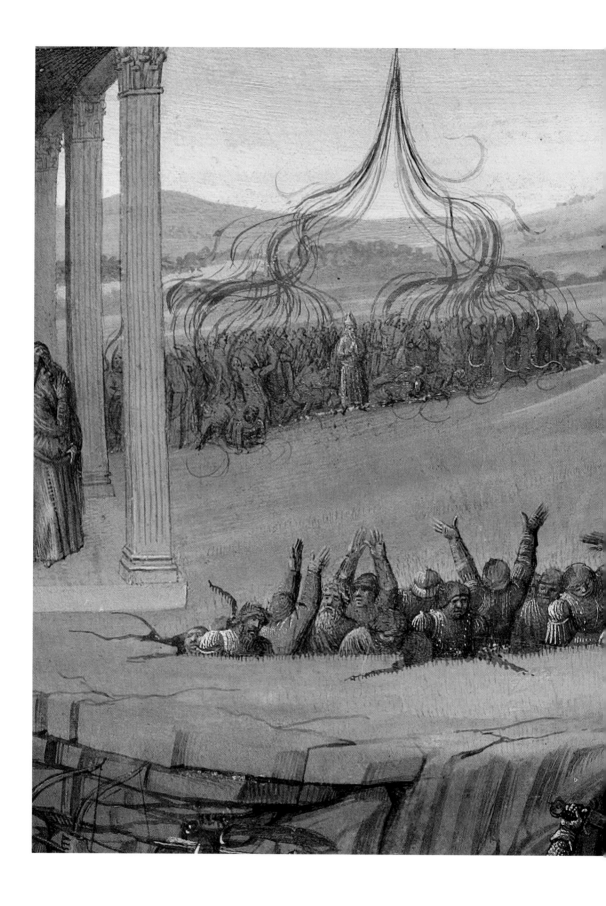

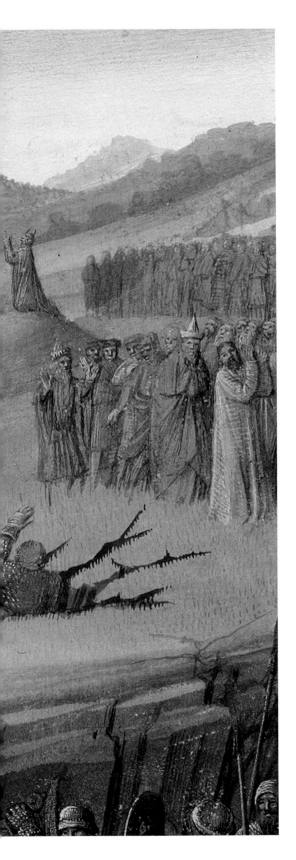

The Sins of the Fathers

Our ancestors' guilt can affect the present generation. The Hebrew prophets show a way out.

HELMUTH EIWEN

IN 1990, MY WIFE, ULI, AND I founded a church in Wiener Neustadt, a city of some forty thousand people south of Vienna. It was hard going; there seemed to be a kind of spiritual torpor hanging over the town. We prayed a great deal about how to respond.

After some time, we felt our prayers had been answered. Through a series of events that seemed to us like divine guidance, we discovered a section of the old city wall in a park, hidden behind shrubs. There we found six ancient

In this illustration from a fifteenth-century manuscript of Josephus' *Antiquities*, fire descends from heaven on the sons of Korah, while beneath them the ground opens up and swallows them.

Hebrew-inscribed gravestones set into the wall; and next to them, a plaque explaining that they were from a Jewish cemetery shuttered in 1496.

Eventually we learned that for centuries, there had been a flourishing Jewish community in our new hometown until the year the cemetery was closed, the year the Habsburg emperor Maximilian I ordered all Jews to leave the city, forbidding them ever to return.

When we read his edict, we recalled the words God spoke to Abraham: "I will bless those who bless you; but whoever curses you I will curse" (Gen. 12:3). Could it be that a curse lay over the city? It certainly seemed possible: the expulsion of the Jews had had fatal economic consequences. Wiener Neustadt had been a flourishing city, but after its large Jewish community was driven out, the city descended into decay.

In the nineteenth century a Jewish community was reestablished, but by the 1930s, with the rise of National Socialism, it was once again threatened and then completely eliminated.

We began to ask ourselves if the guilt of our forebears was still affecting the town's spiritual life, and became increasingly convinced that this was the case. And we began to examine what Scripture can teach about how the guilt of past generations might be healed.

A Curse from the Past?

How can we deal with the "sins of the fathers," the guilt of past generations? Can those of us living today repent for misdeeds committed in the past? In Ezekiel, we read:

> The soul that sinneth, it shall die. The son shall not bear the iniquity of the father, neither shall the father bear the iniquity of the son: the righteousness of the righteous shall be upon him, and the wickedness of the wicked shall be upon him. (Ezek. 18:20)

According to this understanding, people cannot be called to account for the sins of their predecessors, or to repent for their actions. Forgiveness of sins, in the sense of the cleansing and salvation of the sinner, is a personal experience between God and the penitent. No one can step in to be cleansed or forgiven in the sinner's stead.

Yet the Bible describes another important aspect of guilt: the reality that the so-called "sins of the fathers" may have lasting negative results. In other words, even if we do not bear the sins of our ancestors, we may not be able to escape the consequences of their actions.

The Bible describes such negative ramifications with two concepts: punishment and curse. "I the Lord thy God am a jealous God, visiting the iniquity of the fathers upon the children unto the third and fourth generation of them that hate me" (Exod. 20:5). "Our fathers have sinned, and are not; and we have borne their iniquities" (Lam. 5:7).

Such an inheritance may not be personal but collective; God's history is marked not only by relationships and covenants with individuals but with whole groups – families, cities, tribes, and entire peoples or nations.

In Leviticus and Numbers, the negative implications of sin are referred to as a "curse," with consequences on the guilty person himself, his house and family, the group to which he belongs, and the next generations (Lev. 26:14–29, 30–39; Deut. 28). This "curse" is an act of God – he turns his face away from us and we are deprived of his blessing. "And I will set my face against you, and ye shall be slain before your enemies" (Lev. 26:17).

In Exodus 20:5 God says that he visits the sins of his people on their children to the third and the fourth generations. However, this does not mean that after this, the ill effects of their sin automatically dissipate; the curse might be protracted over centuries.

Helmuth Eiwen is pastor of Ichthys Gemeinde, a free evangelical church in Wiener Neustadt, Austria.

A dramatic example appears in the story of Jeroboam (1 Kings 12:28–30). The first monarch of the Northern Kingdom of Israel, Jeroboam set up – in defiance of God – substitute shrines in Dan and Bethel to prevent his people from making regular pilgrimages to the temple in Jerusalem, the city of his political rivals. These places soon became centers of idolatry, the so-called "sin of Jeroboam." This sin had negative results for him personally, for his house, and for his people (the living generation). But it continued to affect successive kings and their subjects, who fell into the same sin (1 Kings 14:10, 15–16; 15:25–26). Ultimately, two centuries after Jeroboam's reign, Samaria was destroyed, the North Kingdom ended, and its people were exiled in Assyria. In 2 Kings 17:21–23, this catastrophe is clearly described as a consequence of the "sin of Jeroboam," a curse inflicted by God himself.

Daniel speaks about this, too, in relation to the Babylonian exile: "Yea, all Israel have transgressed thy law, even by departing, that they might not obey thy voice; therefore the curse is poured upon us, and the oath that is written in the law of Moses the servant of God, because we have sinned against him" (Dan. 9:11). "Because for our sins, and for the iniquities of our fathers, Jerusalem and thy people are become a reproach to all that are about us" (Dan. 9:16).

Two generations later, Nehemiah speaks even more plainly and comprehensively regarding the curse of ancestral sin and the resulting enslavement of the present generation.

> Howbeit thou art just in all that is brought upon us; for thou hast done right, but we have done wickedly: Neither have our kings, our princes, our priests, nor our fathers, kept thy law, nor hearkened unto thy commandments and thy testimonies, wherewith thou didst testify against them. For they have not served thee in their kingdom, and in thy great goodness that thou gavest them, and in the large and fat land which

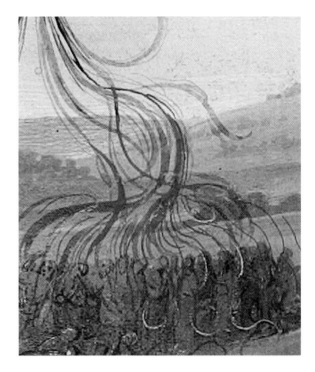

thou gavest before them, neither turned they from their wicked works. Behold, we are servants this day, and for the land that thou gavest unto our fathers to eat the fruit thereof and the good thereof, behold, we are servants in it: And it yieldeth much increase unto the kings whom thou hast set over us because of our sins: also they have dominion over our bodies, and over our cattle, at their pleasure, and we are in great distress.

The ongoing aftereffects of "sins of the fathers" may be temporal: political oppression or subjugation, or economic woe. They may manifest as wars, famines, and natural catastrophes, or as pandemics and plagues.

Just as grave, if less visible, are the spiritual fruits of such sin – the blindness that can lead to unbiblical or faulty theologies being passed from one generation to the next; they may be wrongheaded (and even deadly) traditions, worldviews, and attitudes. Antisemitism is one such malign legacy; its insidious invincibility has poisoned countless souls and continues to do so. Ungodly decisions, stipulations, and legal decrees by government officials or clerical leaders preserve injustice.

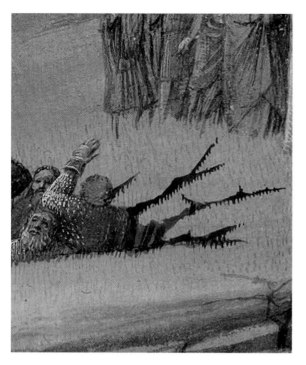

When a dark cloud hangs over a city, region, or a church, its origin does not matter: it will hinder the breaking through of the gospel. More often than not, it will show itself in splits and divisions within Christendom that can be traced back to instances of persecution, hatred, and ostracism.

Repentance by Identification

We cannot repent on behalf of somebody else. But we can identify with them and ask God to lift the curse – the negative consequences – that we are suffering under; we can even be so bold as to pray that he turns it into a blessing.

What does "repentance by identification" for the sins of one's forebears look like, and how might it take place? Daniel's prayer of repentance provides a model:

> I prayed unto the Lord my God, and made my confession, and said, O Lord, the great and dreadful God, keeping the covenant and mercy to them that love him, and to them that keep his commandments; we have sinned, and have committed iniquity, and have done wickedly, and have rebelled, even by departing from thy precepts and from thy judgments . . . therefore the curse is

poured upon us, and the oath that is written in the law of Moses the servant of God, because we have sinned against him.

And he hath confirmed his words, which he spake against us. . . . The Lord our God is righteous in all his works which he doeth: for we obeyed not his voice . . .

O Lord, according to all thy righteousness, I beseech thee, let thine anger and thy fury be turned away from thy city Jerusalem, thy holy mountain: because for our sins, and for the iniquities of our fathers, Jerusalem and thy people are become a reproach to all that are about us. Now therefore, O our God, hear the prayer of thy servant, and his supplications, and cause thy face to shine upon thy sanctuary that is desolate, for the Lord's sake. (Dan. 9:4–5, 11–12, 14, 16–17)

By this token, such repentance requires a double identification: first, with "our fathers," and second, with their sins. Considered biblically, it is clear that God does not see us only as individuals, but always as part of the larger people to which we belong and with which God has a history as well. As individuals, one of the ways we relate to God is by sharing in the fate, the history, the blessing or curse of this people.

What does it mean to be a member of a people? In what way do we claim to identify with those "fathers" of the city whose sins we were repenting? It can be a complicated thing. In my case, my ancestors are not from Wiener Neustadt. But I am a citizen of this city, and we are raising our children here. I have a share in the history of guilt and blessings of this city. I also am a Christian; I am part of the body of believers, some of whom have been guilty of wrongdoing to the city's Jews in its history.

As a member of a people who had become guilty, Daniel was made to personally bear the consequences of their guilt, the suffering of exile, even though he was not guilty himself (Dan. 9:11). It is important that we are ready to identify with our fathers before God the same way. We are bound to them by a common history – by the nexus of past, present, and future. We cannot simply distance ourselves and claim that we have nothing to do with them.

When we identify with our fathers, this cannot be done in a spirit of pointing accusatory fingers at them or, as it were, erasing them from our memory. They are and remain part of the history in which we are bound together by God. Their guilt does not make them our enemies, who are only a burden to us. Thus, as descendants, we are challenged to first treat them with love and respect and to acknowledge that God has also given them in various ways to be a blessing for their descendants. We must be grateful to God for them.

We must also be mindful that it is often impossible for us to comprehend the circumstances, temptations, and influences under which their guilty actions occurred; we don't know how we ourselves would have acted in such situations.

When we ask God in our prayer to cover the guilt of our fathers with the blood of Jesus, we cannot hope that our prayer will be answered if we do so with an accusing and condemning heart. That would be a contradiction in terms.

Daniel was given a clear recognition regarding the sins of his ancestors. He did not seek to remove himself from them, sweep them under the rug, or say they were not his business. Rather, he clearly acknowledged and named sins, and confessed them "before God's countenance." He could do this because he knew he was a member of a people whose ancestors had sinned, and he himself was thus ready to bear the consequences of their sin in his exile – perhaps almost as a guarantor for them.

Nehemiah did the same, saying to God:

Let thine ear now be attentive, and thine eyes open, that thou mayest hear the prayer of thy servant, which I pray before thee now, day and night, for the children of Israel thy servants, and confess the sins of the children of Israel, which we have sinned against thee: both I and my father's house have sinned. (Neh. 1:6)

In such a confession, we include our own guilt – our personal guilt, and the sins of our generation – especially if we or our generation have fallen into the same sins of our forebears. Thus did Daniel and Nehemiah speak – in the first person, acknowledging the sins of their fathers but also their own: "*We* have sinned, *we* have done wickedly" (Dan. 9).

Such a confession implies the recognition that God's judgment and punishment are just. In other words, Daniel and Nehemiah do not complain about the curse under which they and their generation suffer, nor do they accuse God of being unfair. Rather, they agree with God's judgment and acknowledge that the present curse is a just consequence of the ancestral sin in question: "Howbeit thou art just in all that is brought upon us; for thou hast done right, but we have done wickedly" (Neh. 9:33).

Notably, their confession is followed by a prayer for forgiveness and a plea that God might mercifully intervene in the present situation: "Let thy anger and thy fury be turned away from thy city" – its inhabitants in the present generation (Dan. 9:16). Daniel does not pray, "Lord, forgive our fathers, cleanse them of their guilt." That is something they could only do themselves. When Daniel prays for forgiveness, he is asking God to lift today's curse. And so we too pray for God to break today's curse so that the chain of destructive consequences of "the sins of the fathers" might come to an end – and so that there will finally be real freedom, once and for all.

"Cause thy face to shine upon thy sanctuary that is desolate," begs Daniel (Dan. 9:17); this request is central to achieving the goal of what I am calling repentance by identification. It is a request for God to not only lift this or that curse, but to transform it into a blessing; for him to open the door – and even the heavens themselves – to a new chapter, allowing his light to break through our blindness and pouring out the Spirit on us.

Such bold expectation is justified, rooted as

it is in the promise of salvation worked by Jesus on the cross. After all, when he died for our sins, he broke every curse. As the apostle Paul writes, "Christ hath redeemed us from the curse of the law" (Gal. 3:13).

Against the backdrop of Jesus' salvific suffering, we may acknowledge the sins of our forebears before God and ask him to cover them with the blood of his Son so that they are no longer the source of a continuing succession of curses. We can ask him to break that heavy chain, and instead release his blessing. And we can – we must – also believe God's promise that he will truly intervene on our behalf. This is precisely what Daniel experienced in receiving a word that was directed to his people, but whose promise extends far beyond them and their generation:

> And whiles I was speaking, and praying, and confessing my sin and the sin of my people Israel, and presenting my supplication before the Lord my God for the holy mountain of my God; Yea, whiles I was speaking in prayer, even the man Gabriel, whom I had seen in the vision at the beginning, being caused to fly swiftly, touched me about the time of the evening oblation. And he informed me, and talked with me, and said, O Daniel, I am now come forth to give thee skill and understanding. At the beginning of thy supplications the commandment came forth, and I am come to shew thee; for thou art greatly beloved. (Dan. 9:20–23)

A Blessing – and a Task

A confession of identification is a beginning, but to bear fruit, it must lead to concrete action on the part of individuals and the community at hand – to deeds that demonstrate the authenticity of the confession by bringing about real change. Examples might include the correction of false theologies; reconciliation, which encourages new behavior and new attitudes; compensation,

which, to some degree, returns what has been stolen; and the solidification of new attitudes and paradigms by the passing of new insights to the next generation.

For repentance by identification to be fruitful, it must include as many of the individuals and groups who represent the collective body in question as possible. Not only solitary men and women, but whole families, congregations, churches, neighborhoods, cities, and peoples, must be willing to identify with the guilt of their fathers and step into the fissure.

Certainly, an individual can step forward to speak for his family, church, or city, after the biblical examples of those who acknowledged the sins of their fathers – Abraham, Moses, Daniel, Nehemiah, and Ezra.

The work of such repentance can also come about through the initiatives of spiritual leaders; after all, it is they who bear responsibility for the collective over which they preside. Ezra, for example, took on the collective guilt of his people (Ezra 9:1–4). When this occurs, it will naturally spill over and be taken up by the body entire, at the grassroots – in the soil (to extend the image) of a city, region, or nation.

Finally, the secular leadership of a social body (whether an organization, municipality, or nation-state) also has a responsibility to deal with the guilt of its fathers, insofar as they have knowledge that such guilt exists. Though he was a secular leader, Nehemiah confessed the sin of his people before God (Neh. 1:6) and ended up leading his entire people to repent as a nation (Neh. 9:1ff.).

Lifting the Cloud over Our City

It was with all this in mind that we considered the guilt of the city of Wiener Neustadt, once we had learned about it. Eventually, we gathered the leaders of our new congregation and came before God in prayer. Soberly placing ourselves under the guilt of our ancestors, we confessed it as ours, too, and asked God's forgiveness for all the offenses bound up with the persecution of the city's Jews, from the Middle Ages to the present. Then we implored God graciously to turn his face to this city again, and turn the curse into a blessing.

Before long, speaking into the depths of our hearts, God made it clear to us that our internal repentance had to be followed by a public act of external remorse. At a prayer meeting with a group of fellow believers from abroad, one of the visitors reported receiving a vision that showed us a way forward. He said, "I see delegations of Jews from all over the world coming here, standing in this building, beautifully dressed and eating and drinking – as at a celebratory reception. I see, too, a word of God going out from the city to Jews around the whole world."

We asked God to help us discern the concrete meaning of this message, and came to clarity on a course of action: we were to seek out former Jewish citizens of our city who had survived the Holocaust and were now living in other countries and invite them to return to Wiener Neustadt for a "week of encounters" so that we could ask their forgiveness face to face. The vision of such a gathering burned in our hearts, and we asked God to show us how we could make it happen. Through a series of providential circumstances, we were able to locate the addresses of numerous former Jewish citizens of Wiener Neustadt. They were scattered throughout the world, though most had settled in Israel.

And so we wrote each one a letter and invited them to attend our planned "week of encounters" at our expense. The response was overwhelming. In May 1995 we welcomed the first group of some forty Holocaust survivors. Through visits to the mayor's office and to schools, and through other events, the whole city was affected. The focus of this week, however, was an event at our church where we publicly asked our guests to forgive

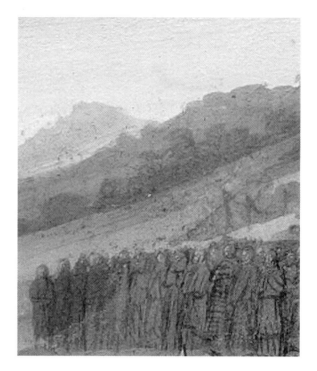

us for all that had been done to them and their families. Tears flowed freely on all sides.

The ongoing testimonies of our Jewish guests after this "week of encounters" were overwhelming. Hearts closed in indifference were opened; hearts previously brimming with bitterness melted. Friendships were forged that continue to this day, although many of the original participants have died in the years since.

One remarkable fruit of this process of "repentance by identification" has been an increased openness to the gospel in Wiener Neustadt. As far as we have been able to observe, God has revitalized not only our congregation's spiritual life but also that of other churches in the city. Many spiritual leaders and congregants gather regularly to pray for revival. I do not know what the future will bring, but I can say this: the spiritual atmosphere has changed, the cloud has lifted, and the skies above Weiner Neustadt are now open to God. ⤳

Translated from the German by Emmy Barth Maendel and Chris Zimmerman.

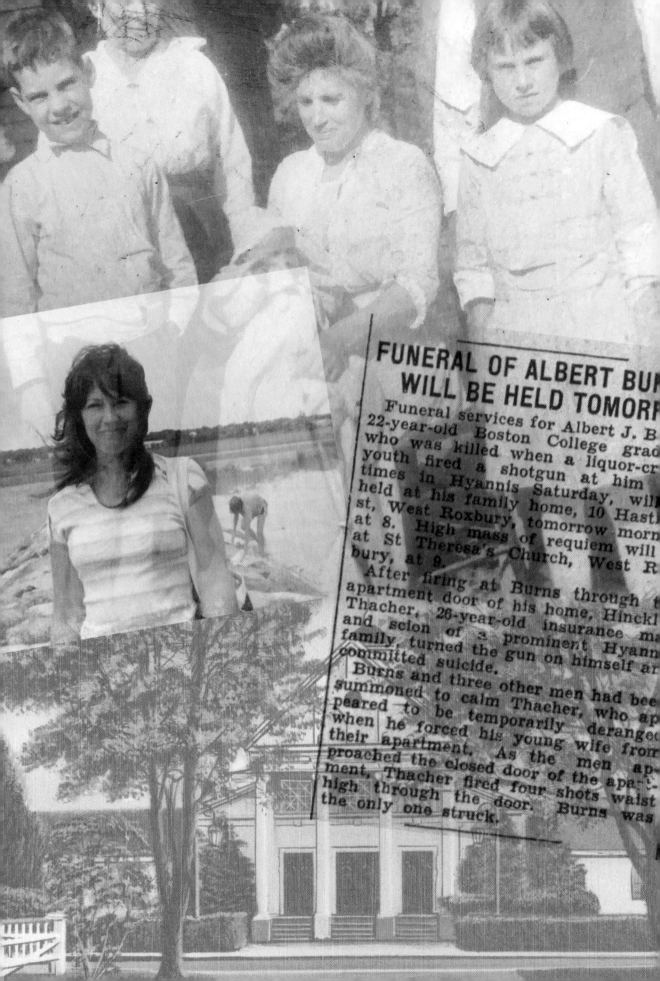

FUNERAL OF ALBERT BU
WILL BE HELD TOMORR

Funeral services for Albert J. B
22-year-old Boston College grad
who was killed when a liquor-cr
youth fired a shotgun at him
times in Hyannis Saturday, will
held at his family home, 10 Hastl
st, West Roxbury, tomorrow morn
at 8. High mass of requiem will
at St Theresa's Church, West R
bury, at 9.

After firing at Burns through t
apartment door of his home, Hinckl
Thacher, 26-year-old insurance ma
and scion of a prominent Hyann
family, turned the gun on himself ar
committed suicide.

Burns and three other men had bee
summoned to calm Thacher, who ap
peared to be temporarily derangec
when he forced his young wife from
their apartment. As the men ap
proached the closed door of the apa
ment, Thacher fired four shots waist
high through the door. Burns was
the only one struck.

Uncle Albert

*An Irish-Catholic family's story of crime
and forgiveness, finally told.*

SPRINGS TOLEDO

ALBERT SEES HER RUNNING across Center Street toward a gas
station with a baby bundled up in her arms. She is a wife
and mother – a wife and mother like his sister Mary, and in
obvious distress. He rushes over to her; others do too. She is crying
and pointing at the apartment house she's just fled. It's her husband,
she says – he came home from a wedding drunk and crazy; he yanked
her by the hair, tried to throw the baby down the stairs.

All heads turn as pandemonium erupts across the street.
A chair is hurled through a second-story window, then another.
A face, contorted with rage, appears for a moment and then a coffee
table is hurled out, a shortwave radio, another chair, pieces of a book-
shelf. The mother and child are quickly ushered into the gas station
under a hail of obscenities.

Albert, at twenty-two the youngest of the men watching the
window, volunteers to go calm the man. Others follow, but Albert
never hesitates. He is one of those singular someones, rashly selfless,
who comes rushing in like the wind where there is distress – the
first to open his hand, his wallet, his arms. Only months earlier, he
was driving in a blinding snowstorm somewhere in Vermont when
his car stalled dead on a railroad crossing. He jumped out and

Opposite page, top: the Burns family, with Albert, *left*, and Mary, *right*; Mary's
daughter Barbara on Cape Cod, 1980; St. Francis Xavier Church, Hyannis.

rushed up the track toward the approaching express train, frantically waving his arms. The train screeched to a stop. The passengers were only slightly jolted, the car only slightly damaged. Albert Burns made page 11 of the *Bethel Courier*.

Albert Burns would soon make page 1 of the *Boston Globe* and the *Boston Herald*.

But right now he's rushing into an apartment house and up the stairs, several steps ahead of a local merchant and a lawyer. When he gets to the second-floor landing he knocks on the door. There's no answer, and no letup to the pandemonium on the other side.

"I'll open it," Albert says. He backs up a few feet, heaves his shoulder against the door, and it gives a little just as a gas station attendant comes bounding up the stairs with a key in his hand. He inserts it into the lock – and a blast from a 20-gauge shotgun shatters the panel. Albert is hit in the lower abdomen. He collapses to the floor.

The others duck and run. Three blasts follow the first; one of them goes through a door across the corridor and destroys an easy chair. As the Good Samaritans gallop across Center Street to the gas station, the face returns to the window, this time behind the shotgun. He fires and misses.

Sirens. The Massachusetts State Police and Hyannis police come skidding up to the building. Four deep, with guns drawn, they enter the house and are climbing the stairs when a sixth blast gets heads ducking again.

Then, silence.

They continue upward, moving warily now, and behold a horrific scene. Albert is lying in a pool of blood across the threshold of the door. He's barely breathing. Inside is the man he had come to help. He too is on the floor. Half his face is blown off, the shotgun clutched in his hand like a last false hope.

THAT HAPPENED IN 1933. "The tragedy in the sudden death of Burns was particularly felt by employees of the chain store where he had worked the past few months," read the next day's *Boston Globe*. "A tall, handsome chap . . . athletic, spirited, and very religious," he was, said a coworker, "as fine a man as I ever knew."

His sister Mary, a wife and mother, had celebrated her twenty-fourth birthday earlier that week. She would never get over his death.

Mary and Albert were Irish twins, born twelve months apart. They were raised in the West Roxbury neighborhood of Boston with Francis, the baby, who arrived eight years after Albert. Their father was a letter carrier whose arthritis bent him, head almost to waist, when he was still in his forties. He was kind. Gentle and kind. Mary and Albert spent their childhoods clinging to him.

Their mother was neither gentle nor kind. After a century of almost impenetrable Boston Irish-Catholic silence, little is known about her and not much can be said. Old records, however, offer a sketch to begin with, a hint perhaps of what was wrong. Mary McNamara was born in the village of Silverhill, in Galway, Ireland, in 1875 and immigrated to Boston in 1899. With no more than a sixth-grade education, she was a servant there and a servant here before marrying Terence Burns in 1908. She was thirty-two. He saved her from poverty-stricken spinsterhood, which was twice the infirmity his was. She may have resented him anyway.

She resented their daughter most of all. Why is anyone's guess.

Two words have slipped through the silence, drifting like dry leaves across a century's span. "Hard" is one. "Unyielding" the other. Images follow: Withering looks. Withering words and blows from a switch. These were brought across

Springs Toledo is a freelance writer of literary nonfiction. He is currently working on a book about the Boston underworld.

the backs and the spirits of the Irish twins, one for the crime of being her daughter, the other because of his insolence – rushing in when his sister was in distress. The cruel mother is an unsettling motif, even today. Motherly love has elements of the divine, but what about motherly loathing – can anything be more harmful to the human heart? The idea of it was too unsettling even for the Brothers Grimm, who winked at innuendos of sex and violence in their collected stories and yet replaced wicked mothers with wicked stepmothers. The original version of "Little Snow-White" included three attempts at filicide and "Hansel and Gretel" turned the sacred image of maternal attachment on its head: *Now their mother led the children even deeper into the forest.*

But Mary and Albert, like Hansel and Gretel, had each other. There was warmth there, and the kind of unbreakable bond that can only be forged in a childhood forest. There was something else. *Someone* else. The Burns children turned to the Blessed Virgin Mary – the mother given to all by Christ on the cross. "Behold, there is your mother," he said to the apostle John, to us. But he beckoned the Burns children – "Behold, *there* is your mother."

The appearance of the Blessed Virgin to three shepherd children her age at Fátima, Portugal, in 1917 held a special place in Mary's heart. She would attend the novena to Our Lady of Perpetual Help on Wednesday evenings and she and Francis recited the Rosary every day of their lives, Mary in her favorite chair and Francis during his after-dinner walks. They ended each decade of the beads with the Fátima Prayer: *Oh my Jesus, forgive us. Save us from the fires of hell. Lead all souls to heaven, especially those in most need.*

Their mother was unmoved by such devotion. It wasn't long before she banished her daughter for reasons only she could understand.

Mary quietly accepted it as she did all things she could not change. On her own and still a teenager, she attended Boston Clerical School,

graduated, and applied for a job at Frigidaire. She overdressed for the interview. Salesman Frank Ryan heard her high heels clicking before he saw the seam running up the back of her nylons. The ice cubes in the floor model melted in her wake, he was sure of it, and so he took a deep breath and approached her, his limp from childhood polio plain to see. All she saw was a swagger. They went for rides in his 1926 Ford and ended up at the altar of St. Theresa of Avila Church, the Burns family's parish. It was March 26, 1930. The ceremony was brief and the guest list thin; Mary's childhood friend was the maid of honor, the groom's cousin

There was only an ancient command – "Bless those who curse you, pray for those who mistreat you" – and the example of another mother, full of grace.

the best man. They boarded with a family across the street from the church, a short walk from the Burns house.

After her wedding, Mary gathered up her courage and knocked on the door. Her mother opened it, frowning, I imagine, like a thunderstorm. "Don't ever darken this doorway again," she said.

Albert was banished soon afterward. He too did the best he could on his own, and his best was very good. He worked at a veterans' hospital and attended Boston College before landing a job in the circulation department at the *Boston American*, a Hearst newspaper. He was representing them in Vermont when his car stalled on a railroad crossing and he stopped a train.

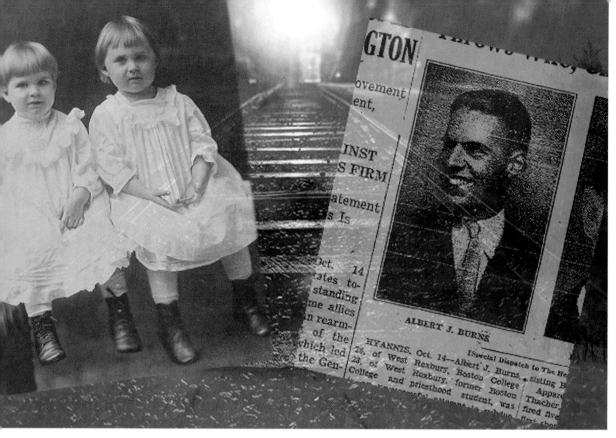

Left, Albert Burns with his sister Mary; *right*, page 1 of the *Boston Herald*, October 15, 1933.

He stood at another crossing around that time, a spiritual one. Within five months, his decision was made: he would devote his life to Christ and become a Jesuit priest. On August 13, 1932, Albert entered St. Stanislaus Novitiate in Guelph, Ontario. There are traces of him to this day: his name appears in the diary of daily activities serving at table, putting up Christmas decorations, attending Adoration during the Forty Hours devotion. We know that he struggled during that first year there, and he wasn't the only novice who did. It was the discipline, the severity of it. The words "hard" and "unyielding" come to mind. An entry appears on February 20, 1933: "Bro. Burns went to Toronto to see Provincial – back in P.M." He persevered another eight weeks before taking a hiatus. The last entry that includes his name appears on April 13.

Albert headed to Cape Cod, the most beautiful part of Massachusetts, where he would recover from the stress and the strain at Guelph. He got a job at the First National, a chain grocery store in Hyannis, and made many friends that summer. Mary was never far from his thoughts. He'd take day trips to see her and the burgeoning Ryan family in Hyde Park, a Boston neighborhood next to West Roxbury. The $25 he'd leave on the kitchen table was a godsend during the Depression years and likely all he had until his next paycheck. He lived his life day by day, did what good he could, and told those closest to him that he planned on resuming his studies to become a Jesuit priest.

He never would. October 14 was hurtling toward him – like blind fate, some would say. Or an express train.

October 14 fell on a Saturday, the day of the week dedicated to the Virgin Mary since the early Middle Ages and the day devout Catholics attend Confession. Albert was among them that Saturday at St. Francis Xavier Parish, receiving the sacrament and the consolation that comes with it at about three o'clock that afternoon. A little over an hour later and a little less than a mile away, he saw a man in distress and went right to him, as he knew Jesus did in the stories of Jairus and the widow at Nain.

Detectives who saw Albert near death on the floor and his murderer's body inside the apartment noted that the door between them had been opened. They surmised that the murderer opened it, saw Albert, and in his despair committed suicide. Were words exchanged between them? No one was there to hear, but had he one more breath Albert would have absolved him then and there, as he himself was absolved at St. Francis Xavier.

Perhaps he did.

ALBERT'S FUNERAL WAS HELD on October 17 – a High Mass of Requiem at St. Theresa's at 9:00 a.m. The wake was at the Burns family home at 8:00 a.m. Mary gathered up her courage and darkened the doorway. Her mother was closing the door on her when she heard her father hobbling toward it. "Now, now! We'll have none of that on this day," he said.

Mary's father died in 1944, the year after Frank plunked down $5,000 for a five-room grand-mansard colonial at 1040 River Street and the year before Barbara, their sixth child, was born. She remembers Mary cooking three meals for nine every day, scrubbing the floors on her hands and knees, beating the rugs with a broom, pulling in a clothesline that seemed to stretch to eternity and back. This was long before front-loading wash towers and microwave ovens. "I don't know how she did it," Barbara says. "I never heard her complain, never once."

Frank wasn't complaining either. When he brought home a Kirby in the late 1940s, she'd vacuum the parlor wearing high heels and nylons with the seams up the back – still melting ice cubes for the father of seven.

In the 1950s, they'd roll up the rugs at 1040 (the family home was always called "ten-forty") for the annual New Year's Eve party. There were sing-alongs with Mary at the piano, a Manhattan with a maraschino cherry in every hand, a "here we go again" performance by a wobbly uncle at the top of the stairs with a towel around his neck – "I'm Superman!"

The house was crowded and the door always open. When Mary's mother got cancer, the door was open for her too. Mary's children remember

---

He never would resume his studies. October 14 was hurtling toward him – like blind fate, some would say. Or an express train.

---

her brushing the Victorian-length white hair of "Grandma," a silent, almost ethereal figure. There's a picture of her taken only months before she died in 1955; she isn't smiling. I like to imagine a moment, just a moment, where she found the grace to touch her daughter's hand and look upon her with love, or something close to it. Mary probably never expected it and may not have needed it, despite modern-day assumptions. She sent a thousand, ten thousand, twenty thousand heaven-bound petitions for her mother's soul. That was how she reconciled herself to what was done to her; there was no confrontation, no catharsis, no copays. There was only an ancient command – "Bless those who curse you, pray for those who mistreat you" – and the example of another mother, full of grace.

Her best friend, also named Mary, wasn't so magnanimous. Barbara remembers hearing the still-fresh outrage of one who witnessed the cruelties. She had barely begun to touch on it when a voice came from the kitchen. "Hush, Mary! That's enough."

The laughter of Mary's grandchildren filled the parlor at 1040 in the 1960s and '70s. I was among those crowded onto her lap as she read *The Wind in the Willows, Madeline,* and *Hansel and Gretel* – the tidied-up version. There were Sunday dinners and Lawrence Welk (I still watch the reruns). She'd play Perry Como records on the hi-fi console and stare off wistfully as he sang "Ave Maria" (I have it on now). By then the Manhattans were mixed, one a day, for Frank in his chair. He didn't get around much anymore and became something of a sitting sage, watching soap operas with an Irish quip for every occasion and circumstance. The Lincoln Memorial reminds me of him. Barbara, my mother, saw to it that he finished his days at home. When he died in August 1984, it was by a bay window and blue hydrangeas; Mary was in the kitchen doorway and heard his last breath.

I was a teenager then and spending more time at 1040 than I should have. My mother sent me there for whole weekends when I got into fistfights: "Don't you dare tell your Nana!" So I'd go in with a bag of clothes, a black eye, and bad explanations: I fell. I fell again. A branch hit me. She must have thought I was the clumsiest grandson in Boston. I was everything Albert was not.

My brother Jeffrey was a different story. On Saturdays, he'd drive her and a host of her friends (all of whom seemed to be named Mary) to 4:00 p.m. Mass at Most Precious Blood in Cleary Square. I was doing who knows what, who knows where, and there's Saint Jeff sitting like an ostrich in a pew with blue-haired Marys on both sides.

One summer day, I poured a glass of cranberry juice and offered Nana the same. "Where's Jeffy?" she said.

"I think he's outside, Nana. I'll go get him for you."

I returned to my cranberry juice. My brother came in.

Her eyes lit up at the sight of him. "Jeffy, can you make me a glass of cranberry juice?"

I think he was twenty-two at the time. Some years later, I came across an old newspaper article about the death of Albert Burns at twenty-two. His photograph was included and the moment I saw it I got something in my eye. I was looking at my brother.

She kept a box in an antique writing desk. Inside was a letter written in 1934 by one of Uncle Albert's fellow novices at Guelph. It was addressed to "Mrs. Mary T. Ryan."

I wish to express my heartfelt sympathy in this irreparable loss of a fine brother (and to me, a dear friend). However, I feel that you will find great consolation in the fact that Albert has quickly gone to his Maker and eternal salvation far removed from the sphere of poor mortals. You should feel supremely happy in that Albert made his long journey away from the cares and strife of this old world completely prepared spiritually. . . .

You must realize that the eventual accident was undoubtedly God's answer and reward to one who had tried so hard to perfect himself, spiritually, against odds. I'm <u>sure</u> that Albert is waiting at the end of the road for all of us who are fortunate enough to reach his destination. . . .

Sincerely yours,
James Murtagh

She cherished that letter. I learned of its existence sixty years after it was written. When she gave me permission to read it, I sat by the bay window with the blue hydrangeas. I asked her a few questions but didn't press – my brother and I had been told that Uncle Albert's death was still a source of great pain for her. We never heard his name on her lips.

Losing him was harder on her than cancer, which she overcame three times – breast cancer in the 1940s, uterine cancer in the 1960s, and

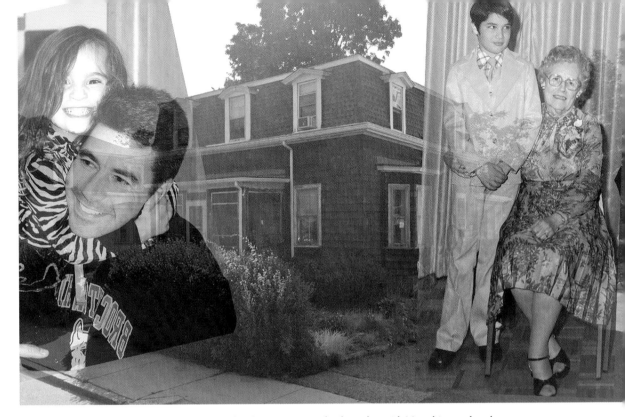

Left, Jeffrey Toledo with his daughter Victoria; *right*, the author with Mary, his grandmother, 1980. In the background is the house at 1040 River Street.

colon cancer in the 1970s. Oncologists in Boston called her "the Iron Horse." When she got up over eighty and could no longer live alone at 1040, my mother took her in. The last decade of her life was spent in Plymouth, Massachusetts, where she continued her daily devotions and buried two sons, including Albert's namesake.

JANUARY 14, 1999, Mary's last day, was exactly sixty-five years and three months after Albert's. It floated toward her as gently as a dove. My mother was awakened that morning by her voice, calling out from the adjacent room: "Mama, Mama." It was before dawn.

Perhaps it's no surprise. As death nears, mind and memory return to the first warmth – to the womb, the first breath, the arms that gathered us up. It makes neurological sense. But science has little else to say and no comfort to give as the body dies. It comes to a cliff and walks itself back. "Show me and I'll believe!"

Faith doesn't need terra firma. It isn't bound by the scientific method because its subject and its object aren't beholden to time or space. It's a whisper in our hearts. "Believe, and I'll show you."

It was snowing outside the window of Mary's room the night she died. She was lying in bed and her hands were fidgeting, reaching, as if for her hat and keys. My mother was nearby and heard her say something that sounded like, "I have to go, I have to go."

There was some distress. We believe that Love Eternal gazed upon her, a favored daughter, and saw that distress.

Whom shall I send?

Here I am, said a familiar someone. *Send me!*

And he came rushing down, as he would. Mary's eyes widened like a little girl's. "Al-buh-buh!" she said. "Al-buh!"

Albert.

And then she was gone. ➤

Special thanks to Barbara Toledo for her memories (and permission), and to Meghan E. Burns and the late Ronald W. Golden Jr. for their genealogical research.

Editors' Picks

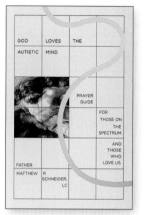

God Loves the Autistic Mind
Prayer Guide
for Those on the
Spectrum and Those
Who Love Us

*by Matthew P.
Schneider
(Pauline Books,
224 pages)*

We need books like *God Loves the Autistic Mind* because, too often, autistic people of faith have been led to feel the opposite. Written by Matthew P. Schneider, a Catholic priest who was diagnosed with autism as an adult, the book takes seriously the unique challenges and gifts of the spiritual lives of people with autistm. Roughly the first half of the book attempts to correct widespread misperceptions about autism: that there's something wrong with people with autism because of their condition; that they're suffering from demonic oppression; that their tendency to be intellectual or introverted or independent thinkers (all personality traits that are common among people on the spectrum) prove maladaptive in a church climate that favors extroversion, obedience, and displays of emotional excess.

This book lovingly and gently dismantles those misperceptions one by one, continually reassuring readers that the autistic brain is good and designed by God. Autistic people aren't defective, they are simply wired differently, in ways that often work to the benefit of themselves and others. Schneider enumerates these potential benefits at some length: the tendency toward having logical minds that enjoy exploring aspects of the faith that don't make rational sense; the propensity to honesty and having a knack for speaking uncomfortable truths; the cultivation of a sense of wonder that challenges others to see the glory in things. These traits, Schneider writes, are gifts to the world and gifts to the church. The most bracing and revelatory portions of the book are those in which Schneider challenges the conformist mindset that sees autism as something to be ashamed of. "Autism is a variation in brain structure, not a demonic influence," he writes. "It is not a spirit to be broken" but a gift to cherish.

He calls his readers and the church to accept the diversity of personalities within faith communities and to resist the notion that everyone must be sociable and emotive. The arguments he develops could be applied to other areas of ability, diversity, and temperament in the church. The church is not harmed because some of its members express their devotion primarily through study. The church is not weakened because some people prefer the familiar rhythms of liturgy over the thunder and drama of contemporary praise and worship. Indeed, they too can contribute to building up the church (Eph. 4:12). Today even many neurotypical ("normal") people are seeking a calmer, more traditional, more reasoned faith; those of us on the spectrum can help lead the way in that. Though prejudice persists, there's a growing movement toward acknowledging the experience of historically marginalized communities; Schneider encourages those of us on the spectrum not to be discouraged by the negative judgments of others while we continue to fight for a faith in which all God's children are welcomed.

*—Boze Herrington,
novelist and blogger*

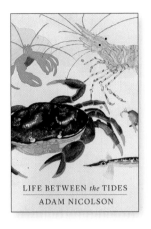

Life between the Tides

*Adam Nicolson
(Farrar, Straus and
Giroux, 384 pages)*

"There are no boundaries here," Adam Nicolson writes about the intertidal zone. "The human, the planetary and the animal all interact, and all of them are interleaved in the realities of the shore. None makes sense without the others." This hypothesis – that the human, the animal, and the planetary can only be understood as interconnected parts of a whole – undergirds Nicolson's latest book *Life between the Tides*. Over the course of a year, Nicolson studies and delights in Scotland's western seashore. Digging through rock and shaping mortar, he constructs a series of tide pools in the Ardtornish Bay. Then he sits back and observes the changes that take place in these miniature seas.

Life between the Tides is a deep dive into shallow waters, exploring the seashore through the lenses of history, marine biology, philosophy, myth, and geology. As a result, the book is many things: part memoir, part field notes, part historical account. The book begins at the micro level: the first section, "Animal," focuses on rock pool inhabitants like winkles and prawns. In the middle section Nicolson zooms out to the macro, considering the shoreline's geologic history and the planetary dance of the tide. He concludes with "People" and the mythology, fears, and desires they impose onto the place where sea meets land.

Nicolson's prose flows from a precise and seemingly inexhaustible quality of attention. A delighted awe energizes the writing, whether he's describing a starfish's arms – "sugar-crusty as an Eccles cake" – or comparing the tide to "a dog nosing in the shallows." Mixed into these poetic and playful descriptions are photos and sketches of the tide pools and their inhabitants, like pages from a naturalist's journal. Nicolson is interested in every facet of life in the intertidal zone, invoking literature and science and philosophy (at times with page-long quotations), with a density of detail that can occasionally stretch the patience of the reader.

The book is a call to know and name the more-than-human world, and to be astonished at the universe contained in something as finite as a tide pool.

He engages in the Adamic vocation of naming. We learn that the scientific identity of a sand hopper (*Orchestia gammarellus*) means the "little shrimp-like dancer," as well as meeting prawns (whose Latin name means "miniscule adventurers"), winkles ("the shorey shore-things"), crabs, and anemones. He gives pages and pages to each tide pool inhabitant, narrating their dramas like epic stories. He challenges notions of what constitutes consciousness by exploring forms of animal knowledge that are beyond human understanding.

Wonder permeates *Life between the Tides*. The book is a call to know and name the more-than-human world, and to be astonished at the universe contained in something as finite as a tide pool. Nicolson's humility before the seashore and its inhabitants is a reminder of our own place in this cosmos. The book is an invitation to practice being with other members of an ecosystem and to wonder at all they can teach us. As Nicolson instructs readers after describing a sand hopper's high-velocity, somersaulting leaps: *be amazed*.

—*Annelise Jolley,
freelance journalist*

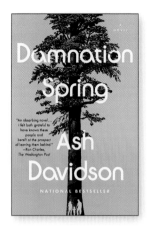

Damnation Spring
A Novel

*by Ash Davidson
(Scribner, 464 pages)*

Beginning near the end of summer in 1977 and chronicling the following twelve months, Ash Davidson's debut novel *Damnation Spring* explores the Northern California logging industry and the generations of residents it has affected. Told through the perspective of numerous narrators, this panoramic narrative offers its readers an intimate look at what it means to care for one's family, one's community of neighbors, and the natural world – and the tension of doing so when those priorities collide.

Rich, one of the primary narrators, is a fifty-something, fourth-generation logger willing to use his lifelong knowledge of the forest to scale redwoods. Colleen, another narrator, is his considerably younger wife who has struggled with multiple seemingly inexplicable miscarriages. In her work as the community midwife, she begins to question whether the logging industry's use of herbicide is associated with the ever-increasing number of miscarriages, stillbirths, and birth defects among her neighbors. When a tense relationship from her past barrels into her present with new information and research into the hidden tactics of her husband's industry, Colleen is torn between her longing for more children and her sincere desire to not undermine Rich's vocation.

As the chapters unfold, switching between narrators in time-stamped journal entries, readers enter into a tale of spousal infidelity replete with dramatic irony, as both characters keep secrets and withhold truths. As Rich and Colleen struggle with the heaviness of real life, some levity is afforded through the occasional narrations of their five-year-old son with his observations about his dog, his bullying cousin, the new world of kindergarten, and the perplexing grownups around him.

Through recounting the quotidian struggles of blue-collar family life, *Damnation Spring* ultimately asks perennial questions: What does it mean to love well? How do boundaries in relationships of all sorts – marital, parental, sororal, communal, vocational – help a community flourish? And where is the line drawn between stewarding your household and prioritizing the well-being of the natural world? These questions are grounded in the concretely political and assuredly controversial topics of logging, shady business tactics, and the imprudent use of untested, manmade chemicals.

Damnation Spring is evocatively written, with wistful storytelling. The use of multiple narrators, a trope often sloppily used, is effectively employed in this case. Davidson's subject matter, vocabulary, dialogue, and characters are Steinbeckian, reminiscent of the ranch hands in *Of Mice and Men* or the migrant workers in *The Grapes of Wrath*, with language just as salty.

This story seems partially to be an homage to Davidson's upbringing in the woods of Northern California. Her knowledge of the land and culture serves her well as an authoritative bard of a fictional story set in a very real place, without feeling either preachy or activistic. A holiday beach read this is not, but when approached as a work of fiction that can make its readers wiser, *Damnation Spring* is effective, and its surprise ending will leave readers feeling unexpectedly hopeful.

—Tsh Oxenreider, author,
At Home in the World

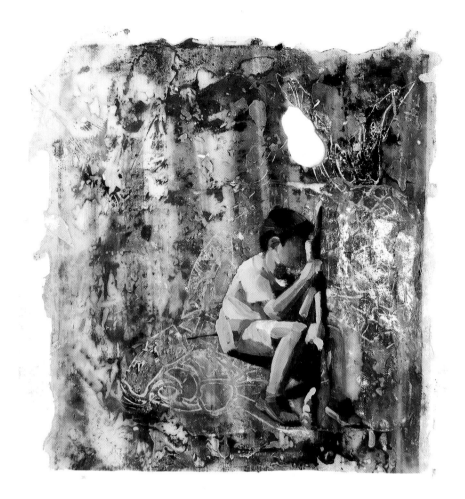

Two Crônicas

A Ukrainian-born Brazilian storyteller remembers
her son and her father in a pair of evocative sketches.

CLARICE LISPECTOR

The novelist Clarice Lispector (1920–1977) was famous for her crônicas – *very short narratives written for the Saturday edition of Rio de Janeiro's* Jornal do Brasil *newspaper. These two have been newly translated by Margaret Jull Costa and Robin Patterson.*

Memory of a Small Son

SEPTEMBER 28, 1968. What to feel about a son? When, in a way, I don't have a single recognizable feeling. What to feel? I see his sunburned face, a face entirely unaware of the expression it's wearing, entirely focused – like some lovely, delicate, fierce creature – on licking an ice cream.

It's chocolate ice cream. My son is licking it. Sometimes this process becomes too slow for his pleasure, and then he takes a bite and makes a face that, again, is entirely unaware of the painful bliss of that frozen fragment filling his hot mouth. It's a very lovely mouth. I look hard at my son, but he's used to my soppy, love-filled

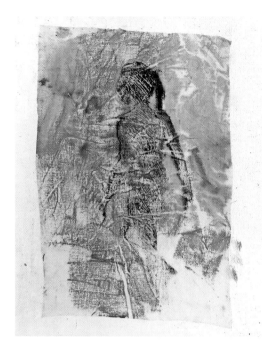

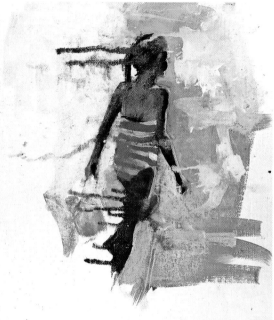

gaze. He doesn't look at me, and doesn't mind being observed in this intimate act, which is both vital and delicate: and he continues to lick his ice cream with his probing red tongue. I don't feel anything, except that I am all of a piece, hewn out of some heavy, fine material, wood of the finest quality. As a mother, I lack finesse. I am rough-hewn and silent. I look with my crude silence, with my empty gaze, at that equally crude face, my son's. I don't feel anything because this is what heavy, indivisible love must be. There I am, in retreat. In retreat from so much feeling. The impenetrable leaves me with a kind of harsh obstinacy; unfathomable is my middle name; here I am, all dressed up by nature. My face must have a stubborn air, my eyes are those of a foreigner who cannot speak the local language. It resembles a kind of torpor. I am incommunicado. My heart is heavy, stubborn, inexpressive, closed off to all suggestions.

I am here and I can see: the boy's face has grown suddenly more intense – he must have found a more chocolaty bit of ice cream, picked up by his quick tongue. No one would call me skinny:

I am fat, heavy, big, with calloused hands that have nothing to do with me but are a legacy from my ancestors. I am a suspicious person who has called for a truce with suspicion. My son is now eating the ice-cream cone. I am an immigrant who put down roots in a new land. My gaze is empty, harsh, keen. And what does it see? A son concentrating hard, eating.

Sea Bathing

JANUARY 25, 1969. My father believed that every year we should all take a sea water cure. And I was never so happy as when we went sea bathing in Olinda, Recife.

My father also believed that the healthiest time to go sea bathing was before sunrise. Leaving the house while it was still dark and catching the empty tram that would carry us to Olinda felt to me like the most amazing of gifts.

I would go to sleep the night before, but my heart remained alert, expectant. And out of sheer excitement, I would wake up just after four in the morning and rouse the rest of the family too.

Bianca Berends, *Sundown Beach Girl*, oil paint and mixed media, 2020.

We would pull on our clothes and leave before breakfast. Because my father believed that this was how it should be: no breakfast.

We went out into the dark street, feeling the predawn breeze. And we would wait for the tram. Until, far off in the distance, we would hear the sound of it approaching. I sat perched on the edge of my seat: my happiness was just beginning. Crossing the dark city gave me something I would never have again. Even while we were on the tram, the weather would begin to brighten, and a tremulous light from the still-hidden sun would bathe us and the world.

I looked at everything: the few people in the street, the journey through the countryside with all the animals already up and awake: "Look, a real pig!" I shouted once, and that cry of astonishment became a family joke, and now and then one of them would turn to me and say, laughing: "Look, a real pig!"

We would pass beautiful horses standing waiting for the dawn.

I don't know what other people's childhoods were like. But that daily trip turned me into a child filled with joy. And it served me as a promise of future happiness. It revealed my capacity for being happy. In an otherwise very unhappy childhood, I clung to the enchanted island of that daily journey.

The day was already beginning even while we were on the tram. My heart beat faster as we approached Olinda. At last, we jumped off and walked to the beach huts across ground that was already a blend of sand and vegetation. We got changed in the huts. And never did a body bloom like mine when I emerged, knowing what awaited me.

The sea at Olinda is very dangerous. You could take just a few steps over the flat bottom, and then plunge down about six feet.

Other people also believed in sea bathing before the sun was up. There was a lifeguard who, for almost no payment, would lead the ladies into the sea: he would spread his arms wide, so that the ladies would have something to hang on to as they did battle with the powerful waves.

The smell of the sea filled me, intoxicated me. Seaweed bobbed on the surface. Oh, I know I can't convey how, for me, those pre-breakfast swims, with the sun still pale on the horizon, were just pure life. I'm almost too moved even to write about them. The sea at Olinda was briny and salty. And I did what I would always do in the future: I put my hands together and plunged into the waves, swallowing a little water as I did: I so wanted to be a part of the sea that I drank from it every day.

We didn't stay long. The sun had already risen, and my father had to go to work early. We got dressed again, our clothes stiff with salt. My salty hair stuck to my head.

Then we would wait in the wind for the tram back to Recife. In the tram, the breeze would leave my hair crisp with salt. I would sometimes lick my arm thick with salt and iodine.

We would only have breakfast when we got home. And just the idea that the following day the sea would be there for me again, made me grow quite serious at the prospect of such venturesome adventures.

My father believed you shouldn't take a shower immediately after sea bathing: the sea should remain on your skin for a few hours. I would reluctantly take a shower later on, leaving myself clean and sealess.

Who should I ask for a repeat of that happiness? How can I feel again the fresh innocence of the red sun rising?

Never again?

Never again.

Never. ⤳

Desiring
Silence

Ancient believers went to the desert
seeking God in the stillness of
open spaces.

SHIRA TELUSHKIN

A SHRIEK OF MANIC LAUGHTER fills the room. I shoot awake, warm in a friend's guestroom just outside Sydney, Australia. The sound is somewhere close, arising then subsiding. Finally the pieces fall together: a mass of kookaburra birds are outside my window, their calls eerily resonant with unhinged human laughter. Soon they move on. Now awake, I go to the window. Sheep-dotted fields slowly reveal themselves as my eyes adjust to the moonlight. Everything is dark and still and beautiful.

I've never liked introduced noise; I seek out cafés that do not play music, turn off my apartment air conditioner the moment a room is cooled to vanish its loud clanging, and secretly hope nobody will restart the jets once a hot tub has ceased bubbling and the night air has reclaimed its soothing hush. I'm the person on the night hike who makes everyone stop for a moment so I can whisper: *Listen*.

As a child I loved the biblical passage where Elijah cowers in the cave on Mount Horeb, fleeing for his life and denouncing his people. I loved how God sends this bombastic prophet first a wind so great and strong it splits mountain rock into shards, then an earthquake, then fire, but comes to him not in these and instead, only, in a *kol d'mama daka*. A thin and fragile whisper, a howl with no sound. A still, small voice. God as a presence we must strain our ears to hear. I always imagined this moment in suspension, like a film when someone hits pause. No warm gust of wind, no buzzing fly, not even the flap of a bird's wing. A perfect stillness. Just desert and silence and (maybe *therefore*?) God. A fragile moment that could be, at any moment, scared away by the shriek of a raven.

It was an idealization of both desert and silence cultivated by a childhood in the heart of New York City, where any encounter with space or quiet was startling, even magical. I'm sure my mother felt the same way. Above her desk in my parents' Upper West Side apartment she had taped, years before I was even born, a photocopied page from an Isaac Bashevis Singer short story, which I read over and over as a child:

> For a while it was quiet. Kuziba dozed off. Shiddah cradled her only son, swaying rhythmically above him. She thought of her husband, Hurmiz, who did not live at home. He went to the yeshiva of Chittim and Tachtim which was thousands of yards deeper, nearer the center of the earth. There he studied the secret of silence. Because silence has many degrees. As Shiddah knew, no matter how quiet it is, it can be even quieter. Silence is like fruits which have pits within pits, seeds within seeds. There is a final silence, a last point so small that it is nothing, yet so mighty that worlds can be created from it. This last point is the essence of all essences . . . this last silence is God. But God himself keeps on penetrating deeper into himself, he descends into his depths. His nature is like a cave without a bottom. He keeps on investigating his own abyss.

This was the silence of my youth: holy, elusive, rare.

Shira Telushkin lives in Brooklyn, where she writes widely on religion, art, meaning, and all things beautiful. Her work has appeared in the New York Times, *the* Washington Post, *the* Atlantic, *and many other publications. She is currently working on a book about monastic intrigue in modern America.*

OF COURSE, FOR MUCH of human history silence was more often noted with fear. In the Bible, people who find themselves alone in dark spaces (Joseph in the pit, Jonah in the whale) invariably do not want to be there. To be immersed in deep quiet meant something was wrong, likely very wrong. "The dead do not praise the Lord nor do any that go down into silence," the psalmist reminds us, equating silence with death. (A not unreasonable association, I was reminded, when a few days after being awoken I passed an exhibit of hanging birdcages, each playing the call of a recently extinct Australian bird, now forever silenced.) Silence was often evoked as evidence of being abandoned by the world or by God. Even worship, in the ancient Near East, was no quiet meditation of the heart but something noisy, loud, often sung or shouted, ideally in a temple.

And yet today, far from being unnerving, silence is usually the soundtrack of transcendent possibility, the sound we most associate with open space. Surely I am not the only one who waxes poetic about echoey galleries with soaring ceilings or abandoned warehouses shimmering with uninterrupted space. And what is more majestic than the desert at sunrise, an expanse of ocean, or walking alone along a forest path densely enclosed by trees? In all these moments it is the unexpected encounter with silence that heightens the experience. Silence is sonic vastness just as a desert is physical vastness. In cramped quarters we are hemmed in by stuff; in crowded soundscapes we are limited by noises.

But what sounds count as silence, and what sounds count as noise? Is silence the rare glimpse of divine experience, or is it compatible with human presence, accessible and available if only we had the ears to hear it?

This is the question Kim Haines-Eitzen investigates in *Sonorous Desert: What Deep Listening Taught Early Christian Monks – And What It Can Teach Us.* Inspired by her work as a scholar of early Christian monasticism, the book is structured around her journeys to capture the sounds of various deserts and remote monasteries across the world, initially to gain better insight into "how natural sounds impacted ancient monasticism." She wants to know: "What did ancient monks hear in their environment? And what did they learn from these sounds?" The book quickly veers from the tightness of this early interest into a narrative reflection on silence, rooted in ancient Christian sources and the sounds of remote places, but also meditating more broadly on conceptions of wilderness in the modern world, the experience of sound-seeking, and desert community. In a neat bit of multisensory innovation, each chapter includes a QR-code link to one of her field recordings.

Though at times more sentimental than might suit every reader, Haines-Eitzen's attention to sound and its impact on our sense of place is impeccable and revelatory. It is impossible to read this book and not rethink our soundscapes.

At the Monastery of Christ in the Desert in New Mexico, she sets up her equipment and soon is recording "the croak of ravens" flapping their wings, a rooster crowing, the buzzing of flies, a prop plane overhead. The sound of nearby rivers and fountains trickles through her microphone. It is the silent cacophony that forces her "to rethink my own ideas about silence as absence. As I listen to the rich sonority of desert landscape, I quest less for silence and more for a quality of presence, and perhaps even 'excess.'"

Her central insight is that silence is a sound alongside others, one we can seek or learn to recognize or choose to cultivate. Silence, she argues, does not require the absence of humans, and it sounds different in different places. Several times she emphasizes that "the desert has never been deserted," insisting on human presence and human sounds as woven into the reality of desert silence.

This thesis is sometimes at odds with the desire for a more otherworldly and total silence she finds in her texts, and perhaps even her own heart.

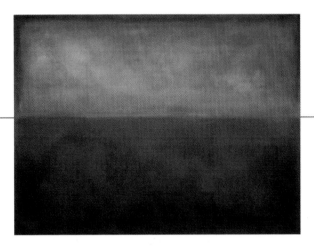

Elsewhere, in Death Valley, she recalls how she began this process of field recordings (for which she attended trainings at Cornell's Lab of Ornithology) "in the hopes of capturing the silence evoked by monastic literature; here I thought I had found it, but it was somewhat tempered: a quiet place for sure, but silence as the pure absence of sound was still elusive." Sometimes she sees this realization as useful for her work. "Slowly and reluctantly, I gave way to the experience of elusive silence, noting that this too was an important feature of monasticism – the desire for solitude, stillness, and quiet was always sought but seldom found."

In another scene, she is in the Judean desert, where she has trekked down the canyon walls to the Monastery of Saint George with her recording gear. "I was eager to record the sounds of the breeze through palm trees, the starlings and doves and ravens, and the brilliant echoes of the canyon," she writes. "But I was also worrying." Pilgrims have begun to arrive at the monastery by both foot and mule, and "human chatter and the clatter of rocks" fill her headphones. Later some monks offer to knock on the semantron, the wooden board that calls the monks to prayer, so she can "record its rhythms and hear its echoes down the canyon." A quintessentially monastic sound, if not monastic silence. Before she leaves the monks gather in the chapel to pray, their hymns stopping the pilgrims in their tracks, as a new sort of reverential quiet fills the room. Though "the monks do not permit pictures of themselves," she finds, "they were warmly hospitable and glad to sing for my recorder." Images might be concerning, but sound somehow escapes this concern of corruption, or unseemliness. Sound is more pure, less rooted in the material drudgery of this physical world. I think of ancient texts that vividly describe God in detailed praise, but would bristle at the blasphemous suggestion that God be drawn.

F HAINES-EITZEN IS CONFLICTED about her desire for total silence, it is an ancient site of conflict. Even in the desert, finding that perfect quiet was never easy. There was always some other monk living more silently in some cave far deeper in the inner deserts, or some bygone era of silence that monks, even in the fourth century, insisted would never come again. In one story from *The Sayings of the Desert Fathers*, she quotes

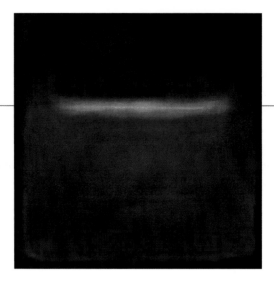

the annoyance of Abba Arsenius upon hearing reeds move in the wind. Turning to his disciples, he says, "When one who is sitting in total stillness hears the voice of the sparrow, his heart no longer experiences total stillness. How much worse it is when you hear the movement of those reeds." Though at times she argues for birds and reeds as sounds of total stillness, "the challenges of cultivating inner stillness in the midst of surrounding noisy soundscape" were not solved by the move to the desert. In this way, the monastic search for inner quiet amidst a sea of noise is more familiar than distant.

And while the desire for silence is often seen as the hallmark of early monastic life – indeed, it was its growth, alongside Hellenistic influence, which finally moved the church to embrace silent prayer – the deserts were not always imagined as sites of ideal silence. Often, the monks saw the desert as a battleground. When Antony first ventures out to the desert, he is assaulted by demons who shriek, roar, thunder, and crash around him like a mob of people. This is par for the course, in some ways. "The sounds inform

Antony's sense of where he is and who he is – he is in the place of demons," she writes; "his hermitage at the tombs was not Henry David Thoreau's idyllic Walden." The desert had to be conquered, more often than not. Even heaven, she notes later, is not silent but full of singing angels and trumpets – and the monastic literature is full of monks who are distinguished in their holiness by their ability to hear such sounds when others cannot. Sound can have its place in holiness too.

It is a reminder that in my own veneration of silence I missed the equally important flipside: In most religious texts, silence is not just about the absence of noise, but the ability to hear something else. The monks went to the desert not just to escape noise, but to find something.

But what?

Haines-Eitzen writes about the popular story of a miraculous camel that stops drawing water when the monks are called to prayer, to not drown out the sound; the machine is disruptive noise, the call monastic. I'm reminded of another early monastic text from *The Sayings of the Desert Fathers*, where Abba Zeno visits a man renowned

BD Griffith, *Fermata 1806,* acrylic on canvas, 2018.

for his fasting but who, when faced with the prospect of working in silence and secrecy (that is, without praise), discovers he is no longer able to fast. Until now, Abba Zeno explains, "you were feeding yourself through your ears." The wrong sort of sounds, filling our ears, can keep us from hearing the right calls, soothe us into abandoning the right fights. In silence, we cannot evade ourselves. "The stories," says Haines-Eitzen, "aren't about noise and silence, but rather about which sounds command attention."

What sounds command our attention?

SOUND HAS ALMOST ALWAYS been the sense over which humans have the least control. We can buy blackout curtains, close our eyes, fill a room with scented candles or sweet perfume, but even the muffled blunted silence of earplugs and sound machines can rarely mimic the vastness of natural silence. Sound, instead, comes at us all the time, in every moment. A boisterous group of friends giggling under our window. A truck honking its horn. The colleague who won't stop coughing. Haines-Eitzen is not interested in noise – there is no engagement, for example, with the growing literature around sound pollution and its effects on urban dwellers, ocean mammals, and the environment, nor with why so many people today seek to live with the nonstop accompaniment of music or podcasts or news in their ears as they cook, dress, travel, run. Instead, she wants mostly to consider whether the desert silence romanticized in religious literature might not exist, or exist fleetingly, but if there is something else there that is deeply human and deeply worth hearing. She says yes, but her case might fail to turn the stubbornly seeking heart.

I think about this as I make my way one morning to the Hungarian Pastry Shop, assaulted by the sheer loudness of the Upper West Side – electric trucks that hum, sanitation vehicles with their huge circling brushes, the beep beep beeeeeep of backing-up vans. Motorcycles. Trucks

full of bread or soda or cheese rumbling down the street. Even St. John the Divine is swarmed with men and their jackhammers, fixing something below the concrete.

Was the city always this loud? Had this book simply made me aware of how little access humans among other humans have to silence? Once inside the coffee shop, people turn pages in their books, spoons clink against coffee cups, the espresso machine grinds its beans. There are sounds, distinct and audible, but they are not *noise*. When a cell phone rings it is jarring, and people glare at the offender. There is a distinct soundscape to a coffee shop, a study hall, children at play. One wonders if the popularity of ASMR videos reflects this desire to tap into, on demand and from any location, the soothing power of specific sounds. Perhaps silence too can be recorded, sought and found, the sonic vastness sought by ancient monks delivered today to our headphones. But Haines-Eitzen's emphasis on the sonorous desert, the silence as soundtrack to this immensity of space, keeps the book rooted in the interplay of senses which comprised the monastic environment, sometimes to great benefit, sometimes falling short.

What I do know is that while I often consider how the experiences of my eyes affect my frame of mind, I give less thought to sound. I know that when I do not constantly feed myself through my ears, I force an encounter with myself. And instead, how easily I have begun falling asleep to podcasts so my thoughts don't keep me up at night.

At one point, Haines-Eitzen describes a class discussion she is leading on silence with her students. They consider silence as expectancy, the pause before something happens, "silence not as absence but as the fullness of quiet, a blooming attention, moments where time slows down." Attention, focus, pause. Silence as a moment suspended in time, where if one holds it and stays in it, not distracted by the boom of an earthquake, one might hear a still, small voice. ⤳

Gazapillo

ÓSCAR ESQUIVIAS

TIZÓN HAD BEEN WEAK for a few days, limping and listless. That afternoon he could no longer move his hind legs. He shivered even when lying in the sun, and there were hard lumps in his belly that made him whine and snap when his master tried to feel them. Simeón filled his dog's water bowl and went to sleep. The next morning at dawn he found Tizón stiff, a puddle of dried vomit under his snout. A few geranium petals and drowned mosquitoes floated in the bowl.

Simeón wrapped his dog in a piece of old burlap and dragged the body out to the garage. There, with some difficulty, clumsy with grief, he loaded it into the van. It took him a while to start the vehicle. When it sputtered and caught, the engine sounded tired, like an old man's breathing. He headed toward the top of the moor to let the scavengers deal with the poor animal. He had done the same with his other dogs, whose names he often recited to himself: Luna, Zar, Canelo, Picolín, Laska, Sol, Perro (there was no way to give that devil of a dog a proper name), Bicho, and Tizón. He liked how the litany sounded and he repeated it, drumming on the steering wheel: "Luna, Zar, Canelo, / Picolín, Laska, Sol, / Perro, Bicho, and Tizón."

The road to the moor was wide and paved with well-packed gravel. It had been built a few years before by the company that installed the wind turbines; he called them "mills" although he knew they didn't grind anything.

Their imposing blades swung vigorously in the wind when it blew hard, as if they yearned to kill passing vultures with a swat. Sometimes they succeeded, and the busted carcasses of the birds lay at their feet like offerings to brutal gods.

When he reached the top of the moor, Simeón veered down a side road that was little more than a pair of faint ruts in the grass. Dry thistles scratched furiously at the underside of the van. When he reached a stand of live oaks, he stopped. He opened the rear doors, but before removing Tizón, he sat down on a cairn to smoke. There at ground level, the fall crocuses were in full bloom, those little plants with the childish name "lose-your-lunch" that herald the arrival of autumn.

It was hot. A few wind turbines moved their blades slowly, like reluctant gymnasts, but the others were completely still. Simeón was so lost in thought he did not notice a vehicle approaching, and jumped when he heard its roar. It was a Civil Guard SUV.

An agent got out of the car and walked toward Simeón, adjusting his cap.

"Good morning, and what are you doing here, sir?"

"Nothing. Smoking," Simeón replied, as he nervously got to his feet.

"I can see that. Let's take a look at this vehicle." He said "let's" although he was alone. The wasteland attracted poachers and unauthorized archaeologists and Simeón guessed he had been mistaken for one of them.

"You can't dump carcasses here," the guard told him, realizing that Simeón was a harmless old man. He used a neutral, respectful tone, as if informing Simeón of a rule he was unaware of. Simeón knew that nothing could be dumped on the moor, but the order seemed absurd to him and went against a lifetime's habit. What would eat the carcass if not the scavengers?

Óscar Esquivias is the author of several novels, short story collections, and children's books and poems. His essays on literature, art, and travel have appeared in El País, 20 Minutos, *and* Archiletras. *He is the recipient of the Castile and León Literature Prize and the Sentinel Award.*

The guard had a strong, vaguely southern accent that Simeón couldn't quite place. He was tempted to inquire, but didn't want to appear curious or flippant. During his youth, his itinerant years working in half the factories in Spain, he had often been asked where he was from, a question with a subtext: "You are obviously not from here."

This guard had a red face and clean-shaven cheeks and a head that made him look almost hairless; his pierced ears had no earrings. He was tall, very thin, and smelled of thick cologne. He had the same urbane, slightly stupefied air of Simeón's great-nephews. Simeón assumed that, like them, this guard would dress in party clothes every weekend, go to a disco, dance, get drunk, flirt, and piss long and hard from the many liters of beer the young people drank nowadays. Or like young groups of friends used to do in the village alleys during the summer *Fiesta del Veraneante*.

Simeón offered the guard a cigarette. To his surprise, the young man accepted it. And even lit it.

"What was his name?" asked the young man, pointing his chin at the van as he exhaled smoke with style, like an actor.

"Tizón."

"Was he a good dog?"

The question surprised Simeón. He thought for a minute before replying. "Yes. Very good."

"You'll have to find another."

"No. He was the last one. I'm old myself and don't want to leave any dog an orphan. The next animal to be dumped here will be me."

"Well, whoever does that will land a hefty fine."

That must have been a joke, of course, but the guard said it in a serious, dry tone. He didn't seem to be a very cheerful person. They were silent for a while, smoking and staring at the nearest wind turbine.

"They're ugly, but you have to admit they're imposing, right?" said the guard.

"They impose," Simeón conceded.

Those metal rattletraps, tall as Gothic cathedrals, forced one to look up to God, Simeón thought – although he wasn't entirely sure God was up there. On sleepless summer nights when the heat drove him out of bed, Simeón had gone up there with the dog to contemplate the stars. But the beacons of the turbines were brighter still, some red and others white, flashing intermittently like lightning or tongues of fire. He and the guard stayed there, under that Pentecost, listening to the obstinate noise of the blades and the hum of the nearby highway.

"Do you live down in the village?" asked the guard.

"Yes."

"Have the summer folk left yet?"

"They've left."

"You're going to have a new neighbor. You know, right? The hunters have hired a guard. He's Moroccan, and he has a family."

"That's good." Simeón finished his cigarette and stomped it. "If you don't need me, I'm going home."

"Call the vet, he'll tell you what to do with the body."

"Thank you. Goodbye, good day."

The guard put his hand to his temple in salute.

AT SUNSET, SIMEÓN DROVE BACK up the moor and left Tizón in the stand of live oaks. The first vulture appeared in the distance before he had even started driving home.

Over the last few years, robberies had become commonplace in the region. Gangs of thieves passed through, raiding abandoned sheds, homes, churches, and chapels. They carried off agricultural machinery, household appliances, money, jewelry, chalices, silver votive offerings, chandeliers – things like that. His village wasn't spared, although there was hardly anything valuable left there. The farmers had all gone, their land sold or rented to people from other towns. In fact, only three houses were occupied year-round: Señora Goya's, Señora Paulina's, and his. And the church – oh, the church! – was almost empty and about to fall to its knees and become a ruin. No Mass had been said there for years, not even on the day of the patron saint, Saint Quiteria. (She was a decapitated martyr: Simeón found it revealing that the local saint had no head.) The archdiocese had removed the altarpiece, including the saint, the processional cross, and the silver vessels, and distributed them to parishes in Burgos, the provincial capital, without meeting any protest. The sanctuary was devoured by humidity. Now its mossy vaults only sheltered four plaster images: Saint Isidro, Saint Sebastian, the Virgin of Lourdes, and a Baby Jesus in his cradle. They remained in the deserted building like four convicts condemned to life behind bars.

Until a few months ago, one thing in the church had still been in operation: the clock, installed and maintained by the municipality, which chimed every hour. But one night someone stole the bell. The thieves must have scaled the façade of the church (which was not very high and full of cracks), levered the bronze bell off its mounting and thrown it to the ground. The hole it made when it landed could be seen in the plaza's paving stones. No one heard anything. That was strange, since the hunters' dogs were locked in a nearby pen and must have raised Cain with their barking; those animals protest at every passing swallow.

Since then, the belfry looked miserable, like an eye with an empty socket. Simeón missed the chiming of the hours and the Angelus. Now, he thought, not even Saint Gabriel visited the village. He used to invoke the saint daily (*The angel of the Lord declared unto Mary . . .*) at the strike of twelve. But that was the way things were. He had grown accustomed to life as a succession of losses. Now the village was almost devoid of souls. The only simulacrum of life occurred during summer holidays and a few long weekends, when the village's descendants returned to occupy their forebears' shuttered houses. Then there were people in the streets, and

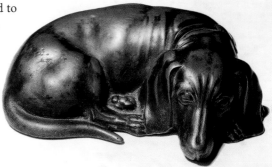

even a festival at the end of August – not the old Saint Quiteria, of course, but a potluck advertised as "the great *paellada*." Everyone gathered in the shady part of the square and ate off plastic plates. Then there were dances that were impossible to follow, and the music blared over a collective drunkenness until dawn. After that, the vacationers returned to their houses in Barcelona, Bilbao, and Madrid, and only the old ones stayed.

There had been only three of them for a long time now: two widows and a bachelor, alone even at Christmas because their children or relatives lived far away. But the three enjoyed good health, plenty of time, sufficient savings, snug houses, gardens, and farmyards. The baker came once a week, the mailman from time to time, the gas man and the diesel tanker when they were called, the garbage man every fortnight, and there was a doctor in Sasamón. They had everything they needed.

And there were the hunters, of course, each autumn. They didn't lodge in the village, though, preferring a nearby hotel. They had legal use of the preserve and had received handsome compensation after suing the electric company for the damage caused by the wind turbines. It was they who cleaned the springs on the moor and installed water stations for the wildlife. They also hired a guard to take care of the dogs and drive them in a minibus from the hotel to the moor.

THE DAY THE MOROCCANS MOVED into the house the hunters had rented, Simeón went over with a bucket full of apricots as a welcome gift. He had waited until late in the afternoon to give them time to unpack. He knocked on the door, then rang the bell and was about to leave when a woman appeared. How unfortunate; he got along better with men.

"Do you eat apricots?" Simeón asked somewhat abruptly.

The woman nodded.

"Well, here you are," he said. When he saw her hesitate, he added: "It's a gift. Do you speak Spanish?"

"My name is Latifa. Thank you very much, that's very kind," she replied, smiling.

"I am Simeón. I live over there." He waved his hand in the general direction of his house.

Suddenly, a boy emerged from among Latifa's skirts like a puppet in a show. He must have been about four years old.

"This is Zacarías," his mother said.

Simeón looked at him silently and raised his eyebrows in greeting. The boy stood still, staring at him with wide eyes.

"Welcome to the village," the old man said. And since he had said everything he had to say, he departed.

The next day, Simeón harvested the apples from his orchard and removed the pitchforks that had been propping up the laden branches. The poor little trees had looked like they were about to walk off, leaning on those canes like old men with crooked backs and a walking stick in each hand. Suddenly, Latifa and Zacarías appeared. Latifa was carrying a plate in her hands.

"For you, Señor Simeón."

The plate was full of something that looked like sweets dipped in honey. They were certainly fresh, because the plate was still warm.

"Thank you very much, Latifa. Here, have an apple. You eat apples, right?" Simeón wasn't quite sure what foods Muslims were forbidden to eat. He knew that they did not drink alcohol (although a Syrian bricklayer who lived in a nearby town was a famous drunk) and that they avoided pork and rabbit. So he wondered if they would avoid certain fruit too. If so, the apple perhaps was one, because of Adam and Eve.

But Latifa raised the corners of her apron and Simeón dumped a dozen apples into it. She seemed very happy with the gift, and thanked him before turning to go. Zacarías watched everything with his owlish eyes. As he left, clutching his mother's skirt, he turned back and stared at the old man the way you look at a dog you suspect might bite you.

But what struck Simeón most was the gesture Latifa made with her apron. She reminded him of his mother, who had died young long ago. She too had carried beans, tomatoes, zucchini that way. And eggs. Like her, Latifa covered her hair with a headscarf and walked with resolution, a graceful way of moving her body that Simeón had forgotten. He felt a lump in his throat. For a moment, he felt like a child again and the word "mother" blossomed on his lips. He hadn't thought of her in years. Now he seemed to see her there, alive, with a toddler who could have been himself nearly eighty years ago.

The next morning, Latifa knocked on his door. She'd brought him another dessert, also covered in honey, heavily spiced and fragrant.

"Thank you very much, Latifa, you needn't bother. Wait there, I'll walk you home and bring along this bucket of apples."

When Simeón returned to his house, he threw the candy in the trash. "Does this woman only make sweets?" he thought. He couldn't bring himself to tell her that the honey would stick to his dentures and pull them out.

Z ACARÍAS DID NOT TAKE LONG to feel at home. He began walking around the village on his own, playing with a stick, a colored ball, or a plastic truck. He chased the cats and was almost like a cat himself, silent and suspicious, wandering here and there. He often approached Simeón and watched him from a distance, very attentive, without ever speaking a word. "*De mal montecillo, bueno es el gazapillo,*" Simeón used to tell him by way of greeting. You'll find a young rabbit even in the most desolate places. To the old man, Zacarías was a sign of resurrection in his beloved dying town, so he gave him the nickname *gazapillo,* little rabbit.

It was sad to always see the boy alone. It reminded him of that year when a stork stayed in the village all winter, shivering in its nest when there was a blizzard and flying through the leaden skies as if lost in a maze.

The guard, Ahmed, resembled his little son in looks and character. He was quite reserved, which is why the villagers – Goya, Paulina, and Simeón – took to him. They had the same disposition and didn't usually trust strangers. At night, Ahmed would smoke one cigarette after another, sometimes a whole pack, on the doorstep, staring at the wind turbines as if hypnotized. Simeón often went out to smoke with him. Sometimes the guard's phone would ring and he would have a long conversation in Arabic that Simeón thought sounded like an argument. Later he realized that it was Ahmed's way of speaking: imperious, emphatic, and bossy. His way of talking in Arabic, that is, because in ordinary life Ahmed hardly spoke. He said hello in the villagers' way, raising his eyebrows, and with that everything was said.

On pleasant afternoons, Señora Goya, Señora Paulina, and Simeón had the custom of bringing a chair down to the plaza to talk for a while before dinner. One evening at the end of September, during the San Miguel warm spell, Zacarías came stumbling up to them. He was more comfortable with the women than with Simeón and even let them pick him up, although he didn't speak to them either. At first, in fact, they had thought the child was mute, until they once heard him cry. Señora Goya, who still had a lot of strength in her arms (she boasted about it), lifted Zacarías up so he could play in the fountain. The boy was caressing the sheet of falling water with his hand when the last rays of the sun flared up, lit the clouds and gilded everything: the houses, the one-eyed façade of the church, the stone fountain, the acacias in the square. Everything shone like an altarpiece. On an impulse, Simeón went to the fountain, cupped his hands, filled them with water and poured it over the child's head: "I baptize you, Gazapillo, in the name of the Father, the Son, and the Holy Spirit."

Señora Goya started and nearly dropped the child into the fountain. "But what are you doing? Can't you see they can see you?"

Simeón shrugged. Zacarías seemed amused by his unexpected bath and threw more water over his little head. At that moment, Latifa appeared in the square, striding briskly. Simeón shrank back.

"The child has gotten a little wet," said Señora Goya as she put him down.

"That's all right. Zacarías, let's go, it's time for dinner."

Latifa walked with him toward home. The others picked up their chairs and left in silence.

WINTER CAME, THE INTENSE COLD, the days with hardly any light. Simeón was chopping kindling when he noticed a presence behind him. Already accustomed to Zacarías' spying, he said loudly, "What are you doing there, Gazapillo, you rascal?"

He turned around and saw the civil guard looking at him from the SUV. This time an even younger man was driving him. Simeón hastened to apologize. "Excuse me, I thought you were someone else."

"What's new? Everything good around here?"

"Everything's fine."

Simeón was afraid the agent would ask him about the dog, but instead the young man pointed his chin at the Moroccans' house and said, "How about those people?"

Simeón shrugged. "They live their lives and they don't bother anyone."

"It must be hard to acclimatize," the guard commented.

"I suppose there are worse places," Simeón answered.

"I guess," the guard replied, and said goodbye.

On Fridays, Ahmed did his shopping in Burgos. He would go to a supermarket by the ring road, then enter the city to stop by a halal butcher and attend prayers at the mosque. He always went alone. Latifa and the child had not left the village since they moved there, and when winter came they hardly left the house. On the evening before his outings, Ahmed visited Señora Goya and Paulina to ask if they needed anything. He also stopped by Simeón, who asked him to pick up tobacco and tinned sardines. That day, as Ahmed entered Simeón's house, he bumped into the cabinet where the old man had placed his nativity scene with its river of silver paper, its Herodian castle, and all the crowded hustle and bustle of washerwomen, shepherds, and other miscellaneous characters. There was a small earthquake. The figurines staggered and some fell.

"I'm sorry," Ahmed said, hurrying to pick one up.

"Don't worry. They're plastic, they don't break."

Ahmed had the figure of King Melchior, mounted on his dromedary, in his hand.

"Do you know who the Three Wise Men are?" Simeón asked.

"Yes."

The old man thought he had said "No."

"They are characters from the Bible, three great sages who knew how to read the stars and brought gifts to Jesus on the night of January 5. Since then they return year after year. Well, that's what children are told, of course. When I was little, people lit bonfires at the top of the moor so the kings would not pass us by. The bell rang out the Magi's special peal, which only sounded on that occasion. Since the village has always been very small, we children were afraid that the kings would forget us and continue straight on to Sasamón. I don't know how they fooled us because the kings were three men of the village badly disguised with painted beards, capes, and crowns made from this and that. But you can't imagine the excitement we felt when we saw them, and how enthusiastically we played the tambourine and sang Christmas carols as we followed them to church to adore the child. One year, my mother was very ill and they came here to our house, right into her bedroom. I was with her. When King Balthasar saw me, he reached into his bag and gave me an orange. I still remember that orange, how good it smelled and tasted, the happiness and comfort it gave me. Do you eat oranges?"

Ahmed smiled. "Yes."

"My mother died the next day. That was the end of my childhood. The orange is my last childhood memory. I was seven. Then there were no more kings or anything else. The sweetness of the world ended for me."

"I'm sorry."

"That's life. The Three Wise Men have not come to the village for many years, and neither to Sasamón. Only old people are left in this region. But in Burgos, they ride in a procession with all their court, laden with gifts. You should see it on Friday, if you have time: the streets are lit up, there are floats in the procession and lots of music. And Zacarías would like it very much, I think. Everyone becomes a child again that day."

Ahmed placed Melchior's figurine in its place. Then he looked Simeón squarely in the eyes, very seriously. "Do you want us to go to the capital?"

"Sure, that's what I'm telling you, go, go. You'll have a good time."

"I mean everyone."

"What's that?"

"Everyone. Zacarías, Latifa, Señora Goya, Señora Paulina, you. We can take the minibus. How many years has it been since you saw the procession?"

"Will the hunters lend us the minibus?"

"The hunters don't need to know anything."

Simeón discussed it with the ladies, and all three agreed it was a crazy idea.

"If my children see me, what will they think?" said Señora Goya.

But later, after they each thought it over, it didn't seem so bad.

"Well, if they see me, they see me."

So they agreed with Ahmed that on Friday, at six in the evening, they would all leave together for Burgos.

On Thursday, Simeón drove Goya and Paulina in the van to Sasamón's hair salon because they said they couldn't go to the parade looking all disheveled. They had their hair permed and dyed. They were glowing with excitement and wouldn't stop quarreling. At their insistence, Simeón also had his hair cut. When he got home, he looked for his suit, the only one he had. He brushed it and tried it on. It was like being back in his body of a few years ago, when he used to dress up and go to the feast of Saint Quiteria and dance in the plaza. He had become stooped since then and put on some weight, but he could still fasten all the buttons. When he looked in the mirror, his former self looked back. He was almost tempted to tell his reflection what his life was going to be like, but it all seemed so sad that he immediately took off the suit and hung it back up.

When he woke on Friday morning, Simeón did not need to look out the window to know that something had happened. Everything was silent, enveloped in a strange light. It was snowing. And that, on the moor and in the village, meant the roads would disappear for a few days. They were cut off. Simeón was downcast.

At noon, Ahmed came to talk to him. "We won't be able to go to the parade. I'm so sorry."

Simeón shrugged. "Poor Gazapillo. He would have enjoyed it very much, I tell you."

"Maybe next time."

"Maybe next time."

IT WAS ALREADY DINNER TIME, but Simeón had no appetite. He had been sad and clumsy all day, bumping into the furniture every time he moved. He had even broken a pretty Talavera pottery ashtray. Its fragments still lay on the floor, mixed with ash and cigarette butts, because he felt too lazy to sweep them up. He sat down on the sofa, turned on the television, and patted the cushion for Tizón to sit next to him. Although immediately aware of his mistake, for a few seconds he had a vivid sense of the dog's presence. Nostalgia washed over him. It had stopped snowing hours ago and the sky had already cleared. Through the window he saw the wind turbines glittering at the top of the moor.

"There's a child in this village and the kings can't stop by today," Simeón said to himself. He rose from the sofa. As he thought about what he could give to Gazapillo, he remembered that in a shoe box were coins he had found. These rusty objects from other centuries sometimes appeared in the furrows after the tractors plowed, and he found them on his walks through the fields. He kept them not because he thought they were worth much, but because, somewhat superstitiously, he used them to forestall swelling when he bruised himself. Pressing the skin with a coin prevented a welt from forming, or so his mother had told him. And as an old man, he continued to follow her advice.

"Children fall and bump themselves a lot," he thought, convincing himself of the goodness of the gift.

He put his suit back on and secured his tie. Then he combed his hair with cologne. The smell of lavender gave him a sudden optimism, as if he were a little drunk. Before leaving, he swept up the remains of the ashtray. Then, very carefully, he walked down Calle de la Peñuela, steadying his feet in the snow as he leaned on the wall with one hand. The snow compounded the moonlight and streetlights. In the square, next to the fountain, he met Goya and Paulina coming down their respective streets.

"The man, the missing one!" they greeted him.

Without another word, the trio started slowly towards the house of Gazapillo. They rang the doorbell, which shrilled loudly.

"That'll frighten them," Señora Paulina said.

Latifa opened the door. She was somewhat surprised, but invited them to come in without asking questions. It was the first time the three old people had passed through the vestibule and entered that house. Most of the walls were still bare, lightbulbs hung by a thread like pears, and there was little furniture. Many belongings and clothes were still in cardboard boxes. Everything looked poor, uncomfortable, and sad. They reached the kitchen. On the table there were a few bowls, some nuts, and large glasses of tea. The boy was in a high chair with his spoon half-sunk in his bowl.

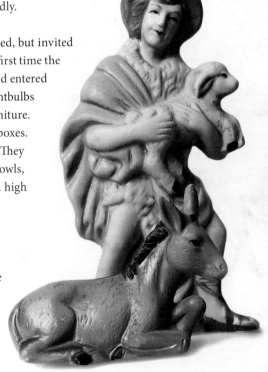

"Hello, Gazapillo," Simeón said.

The boy smiled. "*Hamihala!*"[1]

It was the first word they had heard from him.

Ahmed pulled up some chairs and placed three more bowls on the table. Latifa began to serve a thick stew. It was made of vegetables and chicken

---

1. Old Spanish exclamation from the twelfth-century *Auto de los Reyes Magos*, the earliest extant Spanish drama.—*Trans.*

and smelled of spices and other things the villagers couldn't identify and suspected they wouldn't like, though they kept their opinions to themselves. They began to eat in silence, like members of a family who don't have much to say to each other.

After dessert, Señora Goya suggested that they sing something, because a party without music is no party at all. She prudently began with "Asturias, Beloved Homeland," perhaps to avoid uncomfortable religious allusions. But when she was warmed up, she continued with "To Bethlehem Goes a Donkey" (Simeón joined on the chorus), and then with another Christmas carol, and another. Paulina joined in the last one, although they argued about the lyrics, because one said "*campanitas verdes*" and the other, "*pampanitos verdes.*" They laughed, but neither gave in and their debate got quite heated. Simeón didn't try the sweets dipped in honey, so Latifa offered him an orange. He was so moved he could hardly hold back his tears, but he quickly got over it.

In the end, when they tired of singing, they gave Gazapillo the gifts. They were the most extravagant objects any child had ever received. Simeón's treasure trove was joined by a huge bottle of women's perfume from Señora Goya, and a deck of cards and a green playmat from Señora Paulina, the closest thing to a toy, she said, that she had at home.

The story could have ended here, but it would not be a real Christmas story if I failed to mention that, just at that moment, a bell was heard ringing.

"It's in the church!" Goya said.

"The Magi's peal!" Paulina exclaimed.

The hunters' dogs began to bark excitedly. It seemed their barking came from everywhere, as if they were running loose in the streets. Simeón thought that he distinguished, amid the pandemonium, Tizón's voice. He suddenly felt an intimate certainty, a kind of epiphany, and said solemnly: "Ladies and gentlemen, I can now go in peace. It's a holy night."

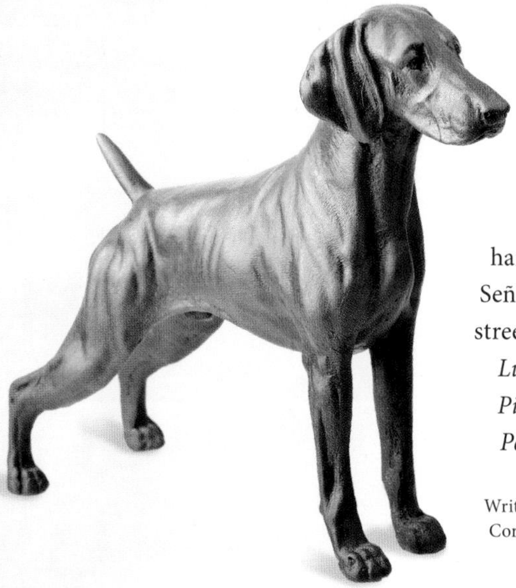

And with haste, as if trying to catch a departing train, he first kissed the child's little hand, then kissed Latifa and Ahmed, Señora Goya and Señora Paulina on the cheeks, and went out into the street. He went toward the barking, saying to himself:

Luna, Zar, Canelo,
Picolín, Laska, Sol,
Perro, Bicho, and Tizón. ⭆

Written for *La noche de navidad* (Encuentro, 2021). Translated by Coretta Thomson.

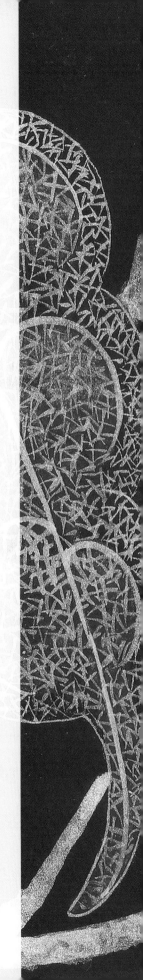

En perseguirme, mundo, qué interesas?

¿En perseguirme, mundo, qué interesas?
¿En qué te ofendo, cuando sólo intento
poner bellezas en mi entendimiento
y no mi entendimiento en las bellezas?

Yo no estimo tesoros ni riquezas,
y así, siempre me causa más contento
poner riquezas en mi entendimiento
que no mi entendimiento en las riquezas.

Yo no estimo hermosura que vencida
es despojo civil de las edades
ni riqueza me agrada fementida,

teniendo por mejor en mis verdades
consumir vanidades de la vida
que consumir la vida en vanidades.

SOR JUANA INÉS DE LA CRUZ (1648–1695)

When You Pursue Me, World

*In which the poet complains of her fate, notes her aversion
to luxuries, and justifies her pleasure in the Muses.*

When you pursue me, world, why do you do it?
How do I harm you, when my sole intent
is to make learning my prize ornament,
not learn to prize ornament and pursue it?

I have no treasure, and I do not rue it,
since all my life I have been most content
rendering mind—by learning—opulent,
not minding opulence, rendering tribute to it.

I have no taste for beauties that decay
and are the spoil of ages as they flee,
nor do those riches please me that betray;

best of all truths I hold this truth to be:
cast all the vanities of life away,
and not your life away on vanity.

TRANSLATION, RHINA P. ESPAILLAT

Artwork: HyunJung Kim, *Prayer of a Cicada*, gold powder on paper, 2017 (detail).

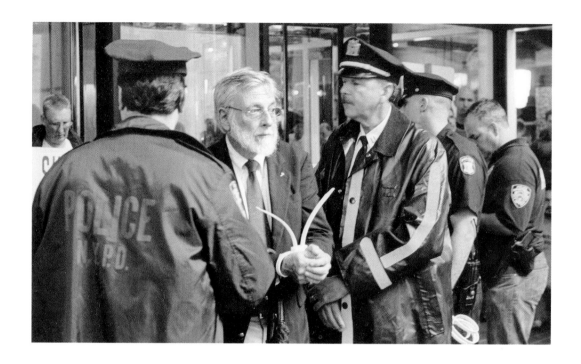

Remembering Tom Cornell

A pillar of the Catholic Worker movement, Tom dedicated his life to peacemaking as an activist, journalist, and Catholic deacon.

FIDA MEIER

O N AUGUST 1, 2022, Monica Cornell called the Fox Hill Bruderhof to let us know that her husband, Tom, had passed away. Tom, a coworker for the kingdom of God here on earth. His was the passion of Christ for the poor that enriched our own calling to live out that justice in the daily life of a faith community.

I went to Tom's funeral Mass, and as the story of his life was powerfully told by Father Martin

Laird, OSA, of Villanova University, I felt immediately drawn into the fellowship of those mourning Tom's passing – the many of us whose lives were touched by his generous care and friendship. Many migrant workers arrived to pay homage to a man who cared, who saw Christ in them – comrades of the road. Catholic Workers were present, along with those for whom they daily make a home, men and women trying to be free of the streets, loneliness, and addiction. Here from all walks of life, we

Fida Meier is a teacher, avid reader, and grandmother who lives at Fox Hill, a Bruderhof in Walden, New York.

Tom Cornell at a protest against Guantánamo Bay, ca. 2016.

were a tight-knit circle, sharing Tom's passion for justice, for peace, for God's rule here on earth.

Tom and Monica's son Tommy welcomed us in the parking lot, and their daughter Deirdre led me to the front to stand next to Monica by the coffin where Tom was laid out, an expression of infinite peace on his face. He wore his deacon garb as a sign of his dedication to the church he loved, in spite of being considered out of step at times due to his radical stand on the teachings of Christ. His worn shoes, which he had claimed from the Catholic Worker donation bin, had taken him down many stony "highways and byways" seeking out and serving the poor.

Monica told me about the three days' and nights' vigil around Tom's bed in the ICU, praying and reading psalms with and for him. He was devoted to daily recitation of his breviary, until at last the faithful heart surrendered his spirit to join the Master he had served. I remembered three such days around my husband Andreas's deathbed, now fifteen years ago. The lines of George MacDonald are a fitting expression for this last vigil:

> And as the childbed on earth
> Is watched by with anxious expectation,
> So the couch of the dying – as we call them –
> May be surrounded by the birthwatchers of the other world,
> Waiting like anxious servants to open the door
> To which this world is but a windswept porch.

Tom had been laid out in a simple pinewood coffin, made by the hands of his brothers in our church community, at his request. There's a story to that, of course.

Invited to a Bruderhof Oktoberfest, perhaps five years ago, Tom and Monica had managed to find time to join us – a rare treat, busy as they were in the daily tasks on Peter Maurin Farm, their home and a Catholic Worker community center. Our pastor, Jakob, another friend of his, then eighty-four years old, asked Tom if there was something

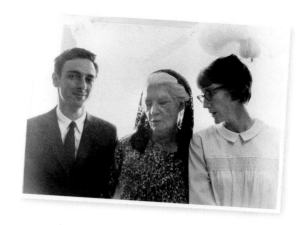

we could do for him. His prompt reply: "Simple pine coffins for Monica and me." They remembered Dorothy Day, buried in one made by the Hutterites. Jakob worked with a young carpenter to build the coffins and deliver them to the basement of the farmhouse, where they stood – surely to the surprise of many a visitor – alongside bookcases containing the many volumes marking the broad interests of these seekers of truth.

How did our family cross paths with the Cornells? In 1982 my husband went through a time of spiritual crisis, as happens in many a serious Christian's life. He took a leave of absence from our community and found himself in Waterbury, unable to find a job as a green-card-carrying Swiss national with no proof of education beyond ninth grade. He decided to at least use his weekends for something beyond his own needs, and looked for a soup kitchen to help out in. There were only two open on Saturday and Sunday.

Standing in the line with many others equally poor in spirit and circumstances, he moved up until he reached the big soup pot and – yes! Tom presiding over it, ladling out the soup, looking each person in the eye. Andreas was taken aback; they had met once before in a very different setting. How to explain himself now? But when Tom raised his penetrating eyes he said with surprise and delight, "We walked together in the Selma March! What can I do for you?" Andreas explained about wanting to help, and Tom, with a twinkle in his eyes, offered, "There are always dishes!" (Andreas was impressed that

Tom and Monica Cornell with Dorothy Day at their wedding, July 16, 1964.

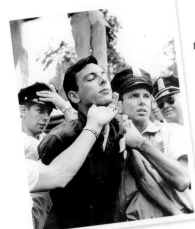

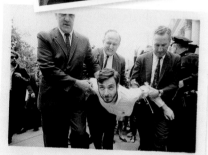

the second soup kitchen was manned by Tom's son Tommy – a teenager whose peers were surely playing soccer on a nearby field while he was heading up a soup line.)

After the long serving line came to an end, Tom invited Andreas to his home, and in the following days, helped him find a job in a furniture shop working with undocumented Latino migrants with whom he found camaraderie and friendship, having spent three years working in factories as a young man in Uruguay.

Tom and Andreas forged an inner bond that held throughout the years. Andreas shared with him his need for spiritual renewal. Tom never probed into details of any personal struggles. He and Monica were simply a loving support in hard times. Andreas appreciated the many meaningful exchanges about the world situation – as well as the signature humor in which Tom clad many personal ills and disappointments, and his dry comments on our country's political leadership and social issues.

On our twenty-fifth wedding anniversary, Andreas told me he wanted to introduce me to some very special people. That is how I met Tom and Monica. Over the following years we would visit once in a while, sitting on tall chairs in their tiny kitchen, savoring laughter mixed with deeper thoughts. It gave us an insight into the other guests they received into their home, folks who had often fallen between the cracks of social

services. One guest came through the kitchen into the living room, talking, talking, talking. Tom looked up from under his brows with a glint in his eye, and compassion in his voice. "The poor fellow can't hold a thought in his head without saying it – from morning till he falls asleep." Yet, he was family.

Another time there was heavy cannon fire in the next room – background to a war movie. Tom, the avid war-resister, looked at us, again with that amusement which could light up his whole face. "What shall I do? One of these guests is dying of cancer. Between appointments, this is what helps him deal with the end of his life. Mind you, I did try a nature film. But it didn't go over very well!" This hospitality moved me profoundly.

I WAS TOUCHED to receive an invitation for their forty-fifth anniversary. Monica was glowing, looking young with a garland of flowers in her hair. She said she felt a little uncomfortable in her new dress (she usually picked her wardrobe from donations and thrift stores). They repeated their wedding vows as a seal on forty-five years of marriage, and in hope for more years ahead. When saying goodbye, I mentioned casually that when the fiftieth came around, we would host them for a celebration at the Bruderhof.

I did not keep track of time, so was surprised by a call from Tom five years later, saying that the coming Saturday they could make it up to our community. And what a wonderful celebration we had, with the Cornells sitting under an arch of sunflowers as the music and entertainment flowed. All of us felt honored to mark this milestone with them.

We thought back over the many touchpoints in our lives. There was the Selma March of March 7, 1965. Like Tom, our community answered the call of Martin Luther King Jr. for a second crossing of the Edmund Pettus Bridge after Bloody Sunday, when the marchers were beaten down by the

Top: Tom arrested at an anti–Vietnam War protest, late 1960s.
Bottom: Tom presents himself to begin his six-month sentence for draft-card burning, August 1968.

home guard. The Bruderhof sent a contingent to Selma, including Andreas. And in Manhattan, there was a young mother like me with a newborn baby in arms – probably also glued to the radio in fear and prayer that there would not be a reprise of the violence, that husband and father would come home safe. That was Monica with three-week-old Tommy; my daughter Francisca was the same age.

Both Andreas's father and mine had served prison sentences in Switzerland because of conscientious objector convictions. Andreas's mother brought her baby boy to the prison, along with some food, so father could meet son. In much the same way, Monica brought her two small children to Danbury prison, where Tom was serving time after burning Vietnam draft cards. Deirdre learned to walk – as Tom told with humor – in the visiting room, though Tommy, then three years old, was somewhat traumatized by the surroundings.

Tom and Monica found their purpose in the Catholic Worker movement with Dorothy Day. Though she respected radical actions in the form of civil disobedience to draw the attention of the public to a wrong, Dorothy Day was convinced that Christ's intention for this world should be demonstrated in daily life. And the Cornells lived out this vision.

I can't imagine it was easy to raise a family while living as dedicated Catholic Workers, supporting networks such as the Catholic Peace Fellowship, Pax Christi, and the Fellowship of Reconciliation, with Tom frequently traveling the country to speak at universities and high schools.

It was Monica, his faithful life companion, who held things together at home. She juggled the donations to cover the daily needs of her own family as well as the family that God placed at their doorstep. Monica created the place that provided Tom with inner and outer care. Both of their children could have turned their backs

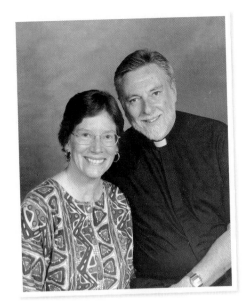

on such a precarious, self-sacrificing life and embraced the American Dream. Yet Deirdre with her husband Kenney have continued the vision, serving the migrant worker community in our area. And Tommy returned from youthful wanderings to take on the farm as well as care for the guests. It comforts me to know that Monica now has them both at her side.

TOM AND MONICA chose a life of practical adherence to Christ's preference for the poor, not because poverty is a virtue in itself (they could see the scars in the souls of those they welcomed, inflicted by the unjust distribution of goods on this earth), but because they saw Christ in them. Together, they made a space at Peter Maurin Farm to demonstrate that other justice – that of the kingdom of God.

In recounting our friendship, I know it only echoes the many encounters others had with them. Tom had an incredible gift to connect with each one on a personal level. All you can say at the end of such a fruitful life is already said in the words of Revelation 14:13: "Happy are the dead who died in the faith of Christ! Henceforth, says the Spirit, they may rest from their labors; for their deeds follow them." ⬎

Tom and Monica, on the one hundredth anniversary of St. Mary's Parish, Marlboro, New York, 2000.

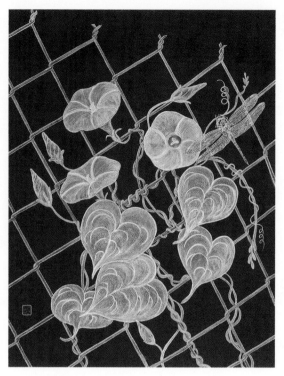

HyunJung Kim, *The Fresh Summer*, 2019

L'esthétique de la Ville

I love when nature recreates the urban.
I love this garden on a fire escape:
water in what had been a fifth of bourbon
steeps lilies; and a cooler, left agape,
holds, over dirt and worms, a swatch of lawn,
a pinwheel and a decorative rock.
Cherry tomato plants are growing on
props sticking from a soil-stuffed cinderblock.
There are some slugs; there is clematis scaling
the brickwork and the air-conditioner.
Plump pigeons, always roosting on the railing,
come for her breadcrumbs. They are tame for her,
the Circe of Gramercy Park, the girl
for whom nibs open and all tendrils curl.

AARON POOCHIGIAN

PLOUGH BOOKLIST

Subscribers 30% discount: use code **PQ30** at checkout.

Members 50% discount: call for code or check your members-only newsletter. Plough Members automatically get new Plough books. Learn more at *plough.com/members*.

Links between Generations

Their Name is Today
Reclaiming Childhood in a Hostile World

Johann Arnold Christoph

There's hope for childhood. Despite a perfect storm of hostile forces that are robbing children of a healthy childhood, courageous parents and teachers who know what's best for children are turning the tide. Every parent, teacher, and childcare provider has the power to make a difference, by giving children time to play, access to nature, and personal attention, and most of all, by defending their right to remain children.

Softcover, 189 pages, ~~$14.00~~ **$9.80 with subscriber discount**

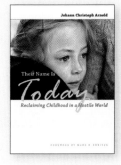

Rich in Years
Finding Peace and Purpose in a Long Life

Johann Christoph Arnold

Johann Christoph Arnold knows, from decades of pastoral experience, what older people and their caregivers can do to make the most of the journey of aging. In this book, he shares stories of people who, in growing older, have found both peace and purpose.

Softcover, 183 pages, ~~$12.00~~, **$8.40 with subscriber discount**

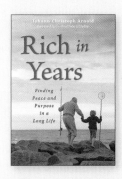

If My Moon Was Your Sun

Andreas Steinhöfel

Did you hear the story about Max, the boy who kidnapped his grandfather from a nursing home? You didn't see it on the news? Well, let me tell you about it.

Max lives in a small town, much smaller than yours. His grandpa is losing his memory, but still remembers quite a bit. Max had skipped school to rescue his grandpa, and they were just starting out on what promised to be one of the best days of their entire lives.

A touching story about dementia and the special relationship between grandparents and grandchildren, with full-color illustrations and a read-along CD audiobook featuring twelve classical pieces for children by Georges Bizet and Sergei Prokofiev.

Hardcover, 80 pages, ~~$19.00~~, **$13.30 with subscriber discount**

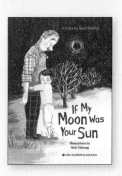

Books for Advent and Christmas

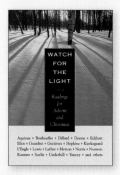

Watch for the Light
Readings for Advent and Christmas

Dietrich Bonhoeffer, Annie Dillard, Thomas Merton, C. S. Lewis, Henri J. M. Nouwen, John Donne, Meister Eckhart, Dorothy Day, T. S. Eliot, Edith Stein, Thomas Aquinas, and others

Ecumenical in scope, these fifty devotions invite the reader to contemplate the great themes of Christmas and the significance that the coming of Jesus has for each of us – not only during Advent, but every day.

Hardcover, 344 pages, ~~$24.00~~ **$16.80 with subscriber discount**

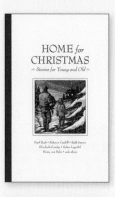

Home for Christmas
Stories for Young and Old

Henry van Dyke, Pearl S. Buck, B. J. Chute, Ruth Sawyer, Elizabeth Goudge, Selma Lagerlöf, Rebecca Caudill, Madeleine L'Engle, and others

"If you're giving one book for Christmas, make it this one." —Jim Trelease, author

Home for Christmas includes twenty time-honored tales. Several are by world-famous authors; others are little-known treasures translated from other languages. Selected for their literary quality and spiritual integrity, they will resonate with readers of all ages, year after year.

Hardcover, 339 pages, ~~$22.00~~ **$15.40 with subscriber discount**

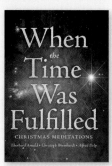

When the Time Was Fulfilled
Christmas Meditations

Eberhard Arnold, Christoph Friedrich Blumhardt, Alfred Delp

The forty short, pithy meditations in this collection witness to the fact that the birth of Jesus is more than history for those who feel their need of him.

Softcover, 166 pages, ~~$10.00~~ **$7.00 with subscriber discount**

STATEMENT OF OWNERSHIP, MANAGEMENT, AND CIRCULATION
(Required by 39 U.S.C. 3685)
Title of publication: Plough Quarterly. Publication No: 0001-6584. 3. Date of filing: October 1, 2022. 4. Frequency of issue: Quarterly. 5. Number of issues published annually: 4. 6. Annual subscription price: $32.00. 7. Complete mailing address of known office of publication: Plough Quarterly, P.O. Box 398, Walden, NY 12586. 8. Same. 9. Publisher: Plough Publishing House, same address. Editor: Peter Mommsen, same address. Managing Editor: Sam Hine, same address. 10. Owner: Plough Publishing House, P.O. Box 398, Walden, NY 12586. 11. Known bondholders, mortgages, and other securities: None.12. The purpose, function, and nonprofit status of this organization and the exempt status for federal income tax purposes have not changed during preceding 12 months. 13. Publication Title: Plough Quarterly. 14. Issue date for circulation data below: Autumn 2021–Summer 2022. 15. Extent and nature of circulation: Average No. copies of each issue during preceding 12 months: A. Total number of copies (net press run): 15,125. B.1. Mailed outside-county paid subscriptions: 11,540. B.2. Mailed in-county paid subscriptions: 0. B.3. Paid distribution outside the mails including sales through dealers and carriers, street vendors, counter sales, and other non-USPS paid distribution: 206. B.4. Other classes mailed through the USPS: 0. C. Total paid distribution: 11,745. D.1. Free distribution by mail: Outside-county: 1,166. D.2. In-county: 0. D.3. Other classes mailed through the USPS: 0. Free distribution outside the mail: 55. E. Total free distribution: 1,221. F. Total Distribution: 12,966. G. Copies not distributed: 2,159. H. Total: 15,125. I. Percent paid: 90.59%. Actual No. copies of single issue published nearest to filing date: A.: 16,000. B.1.: 12,225. B.2.: 0. B.3.: 247. B.4.: 0. C.: 12,472. D.1.: 1,180. D.2.: 0. D.3.: 0. D.4.: 43. E.: 1,223. F.: 13,695. G.: 2,305. H.: 16,000. I.: 91.07 %. Electronic copy circulation: Average No. copies of each issue during preceding 12 months: A. Total No. Electronic Copies: 47. B. Total paid print copies plus paid electronic copies: 11,793. C. Total print distribution plus paid electronic copies: 13,013. D. Percent paid: 90.62%. Actual No. copies of single issue published nearest to filing date: A.: 37. B.: 12,509. C.: 13,732. D.: 91.09%. 17. Publication of Statement of Ownership: Winter 2023. 18. I certify that the statements made by me above are correct and complete. Sam Hine, Editor, September 16, 2022.

(continued from p. 120)

hunger had been fulfilled in – rather than stifled by – the way of Christ.

Augustine, meanwhile, had embarked on a thirteen-year-long common-law marriage to a lower-class woman whom he loved deeply; in AD 372, in Carthage, she bore him a son. They named the boy Adeodatus, "Given by God"; he was cherished. Monica's refusal to accept the woman as a fitting wife for her upper-middle-class son, her refusal to encourage Augustine to make her grandson legitimate, are indications of her own imperfectly crucified pride.

When Augustine finally converted, when the words from Paul's Letter to the Romans like a set of simple instructions gave him the way of life and the will to walk it, it was his mother he told first. "She was filled with joy," Augustine later wrote, addressing God. "You 'changed her grief into joy' far more abundantly than she desired, far dearer and more chaste than she expected when she looked for grandchildren begotten of my body."

But she did love her grandson as well; when Augustine and his concubine parted, to their mutual agony, the boy stayed with his father, and Monica welcomed him into her home. Her prayers for Augustine and (surely) for Adeodatus were finally fulfilled when, on Easter Sunday of AD 387, they were both baptized into the Christian church.

I cannot do more than touch on Augustine's journey here. Monica's own voyage, once she saw her son and grandson into the safe harbor of the church, was coming to its end. She and her son had one last long conversation in speculative theology, at a moment when it was first being worked out: as the astonishing implications of the Good becoming a baby in Mary's womb, of Reason learning to speak at her knee, were being drawn. Standing together at the window of their rented house in Ostia, Rome's harbor city, looking out into the garden, they were "searching together in the presence of the truth which is Yourself."

She came down with a fever five days later, and soon knew that she was dying. She had wanted to be buried with her husband back in Thagaste, but told Augustine not to bother with that – "Nothing is distant from God, and there is no ground for

---

> ## "I cannot sufficiently express the love she had for me, nor how she travailed for me in the spirit with a far keener anguish than when she bore me in the flesh."
> *Augustine of Hippo*

---

fear that at the last day He will not acknowledge me and raise me up." She died nine days after the beginning of her illness, at the age of fifty-six.

Augustine knew that her love for him, her fidelity in prayer, her hope and trust in God had their origins in God's own love and grace. "In her unceasing prayer," he said, "she as it were presented to you your bond of promises. For your mercy is forever, and you deign to make yourself the debtor obliged by your promises to those to whom you forgive all debts."

Adeodatus died shortly after his baptism. Monica had through Augustine no surviving grandchildren. But in an important sense, all those who have converted after reading the *Confessions*, and all those whose hearts found rest in the doctrines of God's grace which he articulated, and all those who have found their household in the church which her son did so much to build: these too are her grandchildren. ⇒

Monica of Thagaste

Her famous son left her no surviving grandchildren.
Yet she became a spiritual grandmother to millions.

SUSANNAH BLACK ROBERTS

ORN IN THAGASTE in Algeria in AD 332, Monica was raised a Christian. Her marriage to the Roman pagan Patricius was difficult; he was unfaithful and quick-tempered, though he could be kind. Augustine, her eldest son, was glad enough to leave the house at age seventeen to go to Carthage to study rhetoric.

Patricius was baptized just before his death, soon after Augustine left home. It was an answer to prayer. But Monica's worries were not over. At school, Augustine, now a long way from his childhood faith, toppled entirely into the kind of respectable debauchery in which many college students find themselves.

He remained fallen away for seventeen years. Academic success, intellectual spelunking amidst the most recondite and fashionable of fourth-century Mediterranean heresies, and sexual adventures were more attractive than fidelity to the Christ proclaimed by Mother Church.

And Monica prayed. She prayed, and she worried, and she hassled him. And she cried. And she prayed. And she didn't give up.

"I cannot sufficiently express the love she had for me," wrote Augustine years later, "nor how she travailed for me in the spirit with a far keener anguish than when she bore me in the flesh."

Monica wanted to take charge of the situation, get Augustine married off to a suitable woman, and find a pastor to talk sense into him. God had his own plans. They took a lot longer than she would have wanted. But she did not lose hope.

She sought allies, theological debaters who could best her son the intellectual on his own terms. This was Augustine, after all: it would have been a tough job. One bishop declined the attempt. "Let him alone for a time. Only pray to God for him. He will of his own accord, by reading, come to discover what an error it is and how great an impiety it is."

This seems like extremely good advice: Augustine was then at the height of his cage-stage Manichaeism, and would have chewed and spit out a standard bishop like a piece of gristle. But Monica really wanted the debate; she wept as she begged him. "As you live," he said, refusing her again, "it is impossible that the son of such tears should perish."

Eventually Monica ran into the future Saint Ambrose, and immediately recognized that here was a man who could finally give Augustine a run for his money intellectually, whose mind, whose own curiosity, erudition, and philosophical

(continued on previous page)

Susannah Black Roberts is a senior editor of Plough. *She and her husband, Alastair Roberts, split their time between New York City and the United Kingdom.*

Opposite: John Nava, *Study for Saint Monica,* oil on canvas, 2003.